Progress in Orthopaedic Surgery Vol. 2

Acetabular Dysplasia
Skeletal Dysplasias in Childhood

Edited by U. H. Weil

Contributors
W. Dega, Poznań · G. D. MacEwen, Wilmington
E. Morscher, Basel · H. L. Moss, New Haven
J. A. Ogden, New Haven · W. Schuster, Gießen
J. Spranger, Mainz · D. C. Stephens, Wilmington
J. Strauß, Nuremberg/Altdorf · H. Wagner, Nuremberg/Altdorf

With 133 Figures

Springer-Verlag
Berlin Heidelberg New York 1978

Editor: U. H. Weil, New Haven Orthopaedic Group, P. C., Orthopaedic Surgery, The Temple Medical Building, 60 Temple Street, New Haven, Connecticut 06510, USA

ISBN-13: 978-3-642-66739-8 e-ISBN-13: 978-3-642-66737-4
DOI: 10.1007/978-3-642-66737-4

Library of Congress Cataloging in Publication Data. Acetabular dysplasia; Skeletal dysplasias in childhood. (Progress in orthopaedic surgery; v. 2) Bibliography: p. Includes index. 1. Hip joint-Dislocation-Addresses, essays, lectures. 2. Acetabulum (Anatomy)-Abnormalities-Addresses, essays, lectures. 3. Acetabulum (Anatomy)-Surgery-Addresses, essays, lectures. 4. Bones-Abnormalities-Addresses, essays, lectures. 5. Pediatric orthopedia-Addresses, essays, lectures. I. Weil, Ulrich Henry. II. Ogden, J. A. III. Title: Pathologic Anatomy of Congenital Hip Disease IV. Series.
RD772.A27 617'.376 77-21579

Typesetting, printing and binding: E. Kieser KG, Augsburg
2120/3321 543210

Introduction

Readers of the first volume of *Progress in Orthopaedic Surgery* may remember the introductory remarks of Drs. Wagner and Hungerford. It is the intention of the editors of this publication to familiarize English–speaking orthopaedists with articles published in the European literature which, because of language barriers, would otherwise be inaccessible to them.

Most articles in this second volume also are translations of papers originally printed in *Der Orthopäde.* The purpose of this German medical journal is to disseminate the newest experiences of orthopaedic problems in a form that is of particular value to the practising orthopaedic surgeon.

In 1973 eight articles were published on acetabular dysplasia. In his foreword to this issue Dr. Wagner stated some of the reasons why such an indepth study was deemed necessary. He was of the opinion that the shallowness and increase in acclivity of the acetabulum was of such central importance in the development and treatment of hip dysplasias that a volume dealing with this subject was fully justified. Another reason for this collection of papers was the advances made in correcting the results of a dysplastic acetabulum by surgical means and thereby improving hip joint function in later years, or at least preventing its early deterioration.

The editors of *Progress in Orthopaedic Surgery* feel that these reasons are just as valid today as in 1973. Therefore, five of the original articles have been selected for translation; where necessary, they have been updated to relate the author's present experiences and opinions. A custom begun in the first volume of *Progress in Orthopaedic Surgery* has been continued: Two original articles by authors living in English-speaking countries have been included; in this volume they give the orthopaedic surgeon an up-to-date synopsis of acetabular dysplasia and its operative therapy.

Hip dysplasias in the widest sense of the term have interested and baffled physicians since the time of Hippocrates. Until the second quarter of the nineteenth century only palliative measures such as braces or shoe corrections had been employed in their treatment.

Ambroise Paré (cit. by J. F. Malgaigne 1840) was the first to observe that the shallowness of the acetabulum prevented reduction of the hip joint, a fact which was confirmed by G. Dupuytren (1826) after he had done a postmortem examination of a patient with congenital dislocation of the hip. His accurate description was actually preceded by G. B. Palletta (1820) who had dissected the hip joints of a 15-day-old male suffering from this deformity. Ch. G. Pravaz (1847) was the first physician who was able to keep the congenitally dislocated femur in the hip socket after accomplishing a reduction.

In the last quarter of the nineteenth century conservative therapy, i.e., closed reduction of congenital hip dislocation, became the treatment of choice after it had been proven to be more successful than open reduction. Closed reduction is mainly connected with the names of A. Paci (1888) and A. Lorenz (1896).

The idea of enlarging the surface of the acetabulum and thereby improving coverage of the femoral head dates back to J. Guérin (1848), who employed a tenotome to scarify the periarticular periosteum around the acetabulum to stimulate bone formation. In 1890 A. Paggi tried to increase coverage by surgically deepening the shallow acetabulum and by reshaping the femoral head. His method was further developed by A. Hoffa (1890). Long-term results with this operation were predictably poor, as it destroyed the joint cartilage; P. C. Colona (1932) attempted to overcome this drawback by his acetabuloplasty. Reconstruction of the acetabular roof by enlarging it with a bony "shelf" acting as a buttress for the femoral head was first undertaken by F. König (1891). This procedure was further developed by F. H. Albee (1915), H. Spitzy (1923), M. Lance (1925), and A. B. Gill (1926).

Surgical reconstruction of the acetabulum can be divided into four groups: 1) Operations in which the acetabular roof is enlarged by a lateral extraarticular bone block to form a shelf or buttress over the femoral head exclusively, i.e., shelf operations; 2) operations in which the roof is osteotomized extracapsularly and then bent down over the femoral head, i.e., acetabuloplasties; 3) operations in which improved coverage is achieved by osteotomy and displacement of parts of the entire pelvis, i.e., pelvic osteotomies; and 4) operations in which the position of the acetabulum alone is altered by an osteotomy, i.e., acetabular osteotomies.

Shelf operations are seldom performed today. G. Hauberg's method (1965) has not become very popular. Indication for the operation appears to be limited to patients in the second decade of life. Our goal in these cases is prevention of further cranial femoral displacement, with the shelf acting as an arthrorisis.

Acetabuloplasties as described by H. Mittelmeier (1964) and T. A. Pemberton (1965) are worthwile and well – accepted procedures in proper circumstances. Pelvic ostotomies as developed by K. Chiari (1956) and by R. B. Salter (1961) have become standard operations. In 1966 A. Hopf published an article on double or triple pelvic osteotomy to improve severe acetabular dysplasia; a somewhat similar operation had been reported by P. LeCoeur in 1965. Neither method has found many adherents. It is interesting to note that H. H. Steel apparently independently developed a basically similar osteotomy (1973). This operation has been modified by D. Sutherland.

In the first two articles in the second volume of *Progress in Orthopaedic Surgery* Drs. J. A. Ogden, H. L. Moss, and W. Dega discuss modern anatomicopathologic concepts of this disorder. Dr. Ogden's beautiful illustrations give added weight to his sometimes revolutionary hypotheses. Dr. Dega's concepts, his enormous clinical experience, and his "supraacetabular and pelvic osteotomy" – a combination of two principles in the treatment of acetabular dysplasia – deserve attention. An article by Dr. W. Schuster gives valuable hints for the radiologic interpretation of the dysplastic acetabulum and contains a timely warning as regards radiation exposure. Dr. H. Wagner reviews femoral osteotomies for congenital hip dysplasia, Dr. E. Morscher discusses some of the European experience with Salter's innominate osteotomy gained on a large number of patients. Dr. J. Strauß reports on observations of patients treated with Chiari's pelvic osteotomy, and the remarkable results. Dr. H. Wagner deals with spherical acetabular osteotomy and the impressive improvement obtained by this method. Drs. D. C. Stephens and G. D. MacEwen discuss other types of pelvic osteotomies and their clinical applications.

Another policy already established in the first volume of *Progress in Orthopaedic Surgery* will also be retained. In a second part, two papers will deal with skeletal dysplasias in childhood. First Dr. J. W. Spranger discusses constitutional disorders of skeletal development. All of us who had the pleasure of reading the book *Bone Dysplasias* (1974) of which he was the senior author will remember his excellence in this field. The second paper, by Dr. H. Wagner on surgical corrections in patients suffering from vitamin D-resistant rickets, gives valuable information as to if and when deformities caused by this disorder should be treated surgically. It is my opinion that the techniques described and the results obtained speak for themselves.

New Haven, Connecticut
September 1977

U. H. Weil

Contents

Acetabular Dysplasia

Pathologic Anatomy of Congenital Hip Disease*

J. A. Ogden and H. L. Moss**

Congenital dislocation of the hip (CDH) is an enigmatic disease presenting in children of varying ages and manifesting as extremely variable deformities that may affect both the acetabulum and proximal femur. The term "dislocation" is not totally appropriate to an adequate concept of CDH. Leveuf emphasized that CDH should be divided into two distinct categories – subluxation and luxation. According to his criteria the acetabular rim is forced superiorly (everted) against the ilium in subluxation, while the rim is inverted into the true acetabulum in a luxation, or true dislocation (Fig. 1). Leveuf referred to the acetabular rim as the

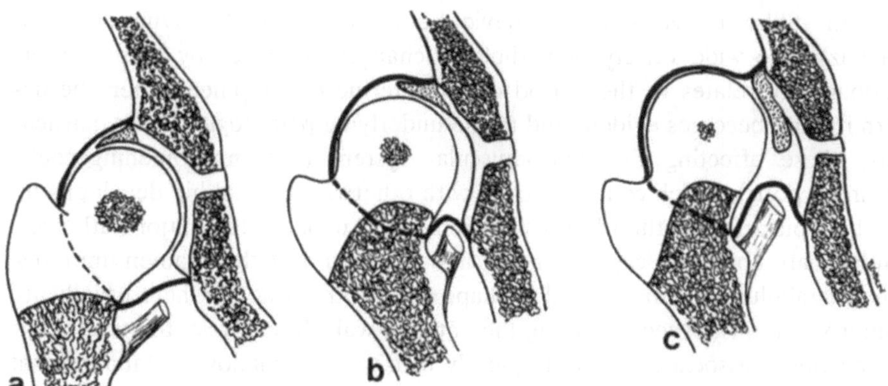

Fig. 1. Schematic drawing of a normal hip (a) and two types of CDH described by Leveuf: subluxation (b) with eversion of the acetabular margin and luxation (c) with inversion of the acetabular margin

limbus, in both the normal hip and the two types of CDH, although prevailing use of the term "limbus" seems confined to the pathologically hypertrophied, inverted acetabular margin of the complete dislocation. As demonstrated by Ogden (1974), the fibrocartilaginous acetabular rim is grossly and histologically

* Departments of Surgery (Orthopaedics) and Pediatrics, and the Human Growth and Development Study Unit, Yale University School of Medicine, New Haven, Connecticut 06510, USA
** Supported in part by grants from the Crippled Children's Aid Society, the Easter Seal Research Foundation, and NIH Grant 1 R01 HD10854

distinct from the hyaline cartilage of the acetabulum, and this marginal tissue is easily deformed by applied pressure, whether acute or chronic.

Congenital hip disease should be viewed as a protean condition that may result from many causes capable of inducing pathologic changes during the intrauterine (fetal) period, the neonatal period (especially during or shortly after childbirth), or during infancy and childhood. The pathologic changes may include acetabular deformity, femoral anteversion, subluxation, complete dislocation and formation of a false acetabulum. The acetabular rim may be everted or inverted. The primary etiologic factors, which appear to be mechanical and physiologic, and the time span of action of these factors control the anatomic changes characteristic of CDH. The reversibility of both the primary causal factors and the secondary pathologic changes will ultimately affect the results of treatment. It is imperative for the orthopaedist to approach each involved patient with a rational evaluation which includes defining, as much as possible, the primary cause and the specific pathologic anatomy.

Studies of the pathologic anatomy of CDH are infrequent, and primarily confined to museum specimens (Fairbank) or hips removed from prenatal or fullterm stillborns (Dega; Stanisavljevic; Laurenson; McKibbin; Dunn; Campos da Paz). The wide variety of pathologic changes described by these authors undoubtedly relates to the period of intrauterine development when the deformity first becomes evident and to the underlying pathologic factors, particularly those affecting the neuromuscular system (e.g. myelomeningocoele, arthrogryposis), which could interfere with otherwise normal hip development. In the typical (idiopathic) hip dislocation in the neonate the major pathologic findings are abnormal capsular laxity and elongation of the ligamentum teres. The acetabulum may be normal in shape and depth, although there usually are minor variations, especially along the anterior wall. In contrast, the teratologic dislocation is associated more frequently with a small, shallow acetabulum that has undergone significant deformation during the intrauterine period. The acetabulum is often filled with a vascular, fibrofatty areolar tissue. The ligamentum teres may be elongated and hypertrophied. The distended posterior capsule may be adherent to the femoral head or the ilium. There may be major distortions of the contour of the femoral head, and the proximal femur may be anteverted. While these changes are more characteristic of the teratologic dislocation, they also may be found in the more severely involved typical (idiopathic) cases.

Specimens of pathologic anatomy from the postnatal growth period are extremely rare (Dega; Ogden and Jensen; Milgram and Tachdjian). During this period the untreated "typical" case may progress from a subluxation to a complete dislocation, developing many of the severe secondary changes associated with the terotologic hip. The mild teratologic hip of a child with myelomeningocoele may also progress. Acquired neurologic disorders (such as cerebral palsy) may cause progressive subluxation and eventual dislocation of previously normal hips.

This paper presents an array of pathologic hip joint deformities representing both typical and teratologic changes, with emphasis on the variability of change and the potential problems that might be encountered during treatment. Concomitant with the presentation of the pathologic material will be an elaboration upon the interrelationships between primary etiologic factors and secondary anatomic changes.

The Intrauterine Period

Congenital hip disease, a highly variable entity, is frequently referred to as a "dysplasia", a term that connotes anatomic malformation. A true congenital malformation is a structural change arising during the embryonic period of organogenesis (prior to eight weeks of gestation) and represents a major alteration of the involved organ system (in this case, the musculoskeletal system). However, with the exception of rare entities such as femoral duplication, proximal femoral focal deficiency and phocomelia, true biologic malformations affecting the hip joint are rare. To better understand the changes affecting the hip, Dunn (1976a) introduced the concept of "congenital deformation", which may be defined as the progressive deformation of a previously normally formed structure during the subsequent fetal period, rather than during the embryonic period. In his eyperience most "deformities" arising after the embryonic period involve the musculoskeletal system and appear to be influenced significantly by intrauterine factors, particularly those which place abnormal mechanical stress on components of the musculoskeletal system. The same phenomenon of gradual deformation may also occur postnatally (especially during the neonatal period), when extrinsic, as well as intrinsic, mechanical factors again may act adversely on a hip that is either normal or has been rendered susceptible to instability by prevailing intrauterine conditions.

Dunn stipulates that gentle mechanical forces, if persistently applied, may lead to gradual, but progressive deformation, and that such deformation occurs much more readily in periods of excessively rapid growth. The fetus is thus particularly susceptible to deformation because of the rapid rate of growth and the relative plasticity of the chondroosseous skeleton. Prenatal deforming forces may be intrinsic (position of the skeletal components, muscle imbalance) or extrinsic (intrauterine muscle tone, amount of amniotic fluid, presence of more than one fetus). The extrinsic forces become more prevalent during the last trimester due to increasing fetal size and a relative decrease in the amniotic fluid volume. As the fetus grows, it becomes increasingly exposed to pressure from the uterine musculature, the maternal spinal column, and the maternal abdominal wall. During this period of development the skeletal system gradually becomes less plastic and more able to resist deformation, although the hip capsule is an exception as it may be altered physicochemically by maternal hormonal changes of the last trimester of pregnancy. The fetus is also developing neuromuscular activity that enables it to kick, change position, and alter alignment along which potentially deforming forces might act.

Congenital hip disease is much more common in the *first* pregnancy. The most important factor appears to be the tight maternal abdominal and uterine musculature, which tends to increase the compressive stresses on the amniotic sac and fetus. In each subsequent pregnancy a certain amount of this muscular tone is lost, thus diminishing some of the extrinsic deforming force.

The breech position also has a high association with congenital hip disease. This position seems to predispose the hip to CDH through two major biomechanical factors. First, the fetal pelvis is held securely in the maternal pelvis, forcing the fetus into an extreme degree of hip flexion, which uncovers a significant portion of the femoral head and leads to capsular distension. In most instances the knees are extended, or even hyperextended. This increases intramuscular forces within the hamstrings, and it may be the most important mechanical factor. Experimentally it has been shown that subluxation and dislocation of the hip may be produced in the rabbit simply by taking a neonatal animal and placing the normally flexed knee in a permanently extended position; this led to a gradual but progressive displacement of the proximal femur from the acetabulum and created a multitude of variations of CDH, ranging from subluxation to complete dislocation (Michellson). Second, the breech position makes it almost impossible for the fetus to kick and to change its position. Without any significant hip motion, the fetus is unable to bring the hip out of this highly susceptible position. This increases the constancy of deforming forces on the biologically plastic acetabular rim and may be the primary cause of the narrowing of the anterior acetabular wall and the contour change from a round acetabulum to an elongated one (this change in shape will be discussed in more detail and illustrated in a subsequent section). The fact that the breech position causes intrauterine dislocation has been fortuitously demonstrated by roentgenography prior to a Caesarian section (Fig. 2).

The volume of amniotic fluid also seems to play a major role among the multiple factors contributing to the etiology of CDH. Dunn (1976a) has demonstrated a strongly positive correlation between oligohydramnios and various kinds of congenital deformations. In sharp contrast, fetuses with congenital (intrauterine postural) deformations never had associated polyhydramnios. Furthermore, when there was premature rupture of the membranes or prolongation of labor, the fetus generally presented with structural deformation. Of 11 fetuses associated with oligohydramnios, Dunn found CDH in six. Oligohydramnios is also frequently associated with urinary tract abnormalities that prevent fetal urination, a condition termed "Potter's syndrome"; these infants also have a high degree of CDH. The amniotic fluid hydrostatically protects the fetus from the mechanical forces of the uterine musculature during the first and second trimesters, when the musculoskeletal system is extremely plastic. Any decrease in the amount of amniotic fluid may increase the susceptibility of the fetus to deforming forces, and may lead to structural changes even during early fetal stages, as will be illustrated by the following case:

This fetus of approximately 22–24 weeks gestation and weighing 2000 g was found to have polycystic kidneys. Examination of the pelvis showed that one acetabulum was

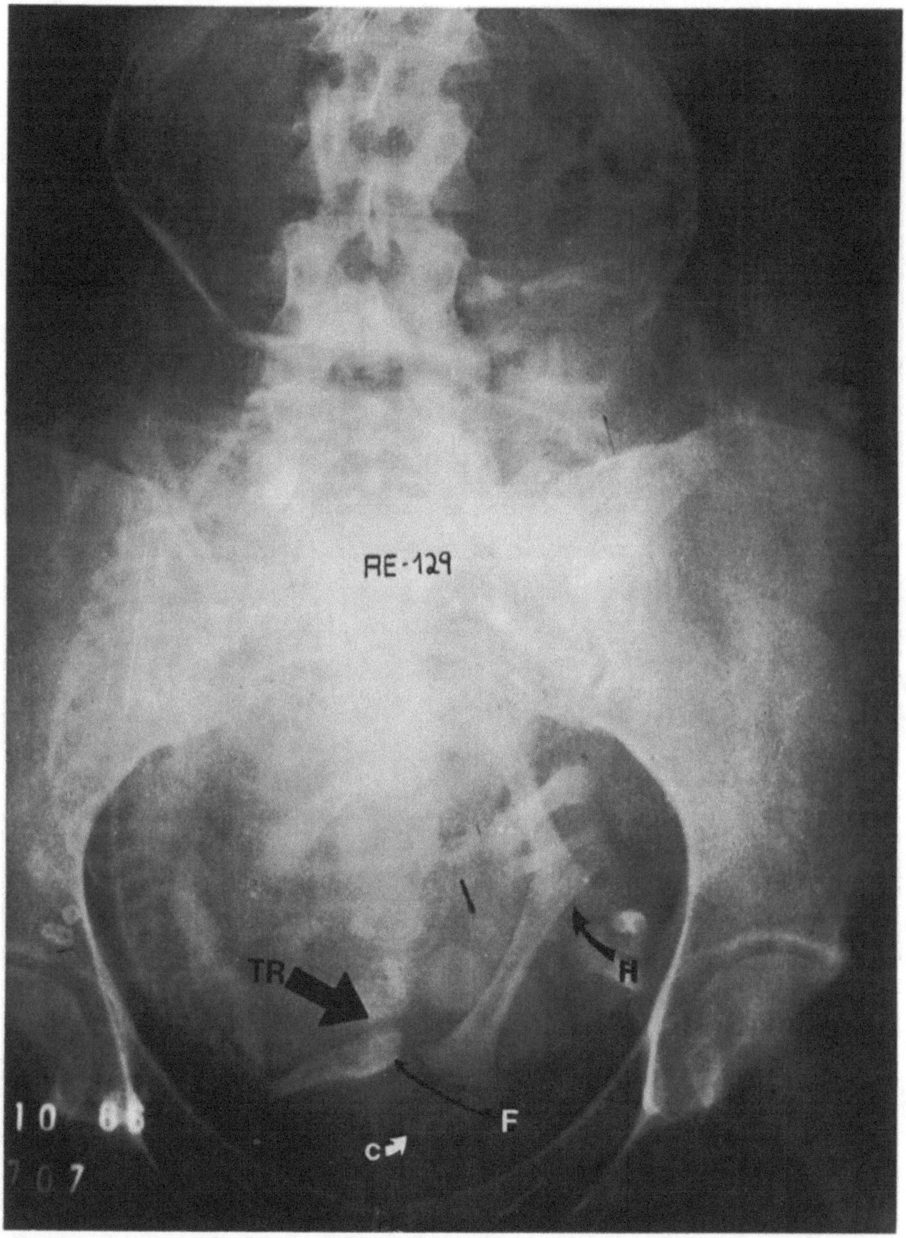

Fig. 2. Prenatal KUB showing breech position of fetus and obvious dislocated hip. The child was found to have CDH during neonatal examination. *TR* – triradiate cartilage; *F* – proximal femur; *C* – capsular distension; *H* – hyperextended knee (roentgenogram courtesy Dr. Aloysio Campos da Paz, Brasilia, Brazil)

normal, while the other had significant deformation (Fig. 3). The abnormal acetabulum was shallow. The rim showed marginal hypertrophy anteriorly and posteriorly, while the superior portion was everted. Interestingly, there was a narrow rim of hypertrophy along the junction of the labrum and hyaline acetabular cartilage superiorly, suggestive of beginning "inversion" of a portion of the labrum. The transverse ligament was hypertrophic and covered a part of the inferior acetabulum. The capsule was densely adherent to the everted portion of the labrum, in sharp contrast to the normal state, in which these two structures may be easily separated. A roentgenogram of the pelvis showed that the ossifying portions of the iliac bones were symmetric and appeared to have a normal index, despite the fact that there was an obvious difference in the shape of the cartilaginous components of the affected acetabulum.

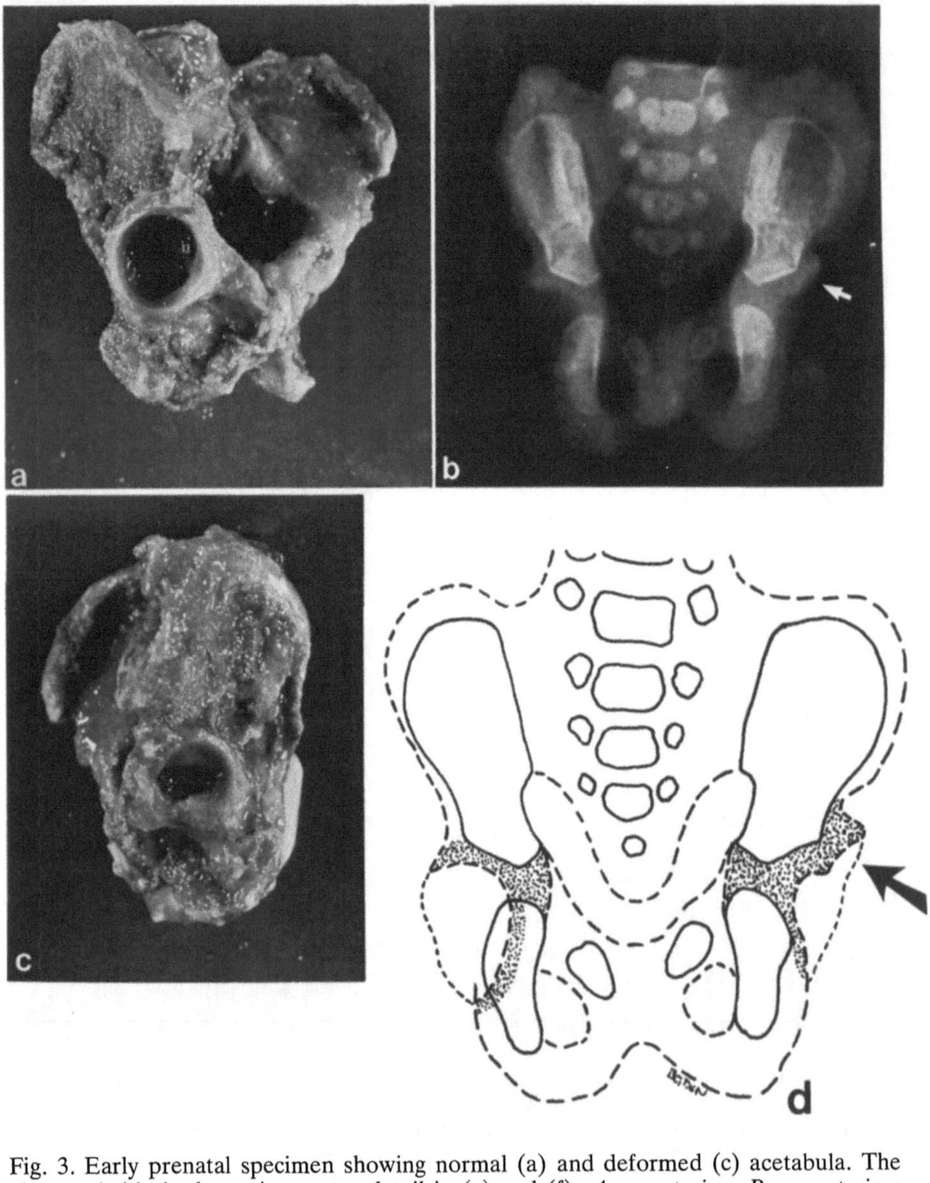

Fig. 3. Early prenatal specimen showing normal (a) and deformed (c) acetabula. The abnormal side is shown in greater detail in (e) and (f); *A* – anterior; *P* – posterior; *IP* – indentation of anterior wall of acetabulum made by iliopsoas and anteverted femoral head; *LCF* – ligamentum capitum femoris. There was a grossly obvious inverted labrum (limbus), but there was associated eversion of adjacent portions. Sections (b) and (d) show the roentgenogram of the specimen. The osseous roof of the acetabulum is symmetric and has a normal acclivity, despite the obvious cartilaginous deformity. The acetabular cartilage is stippled in the schematic drawing (d)

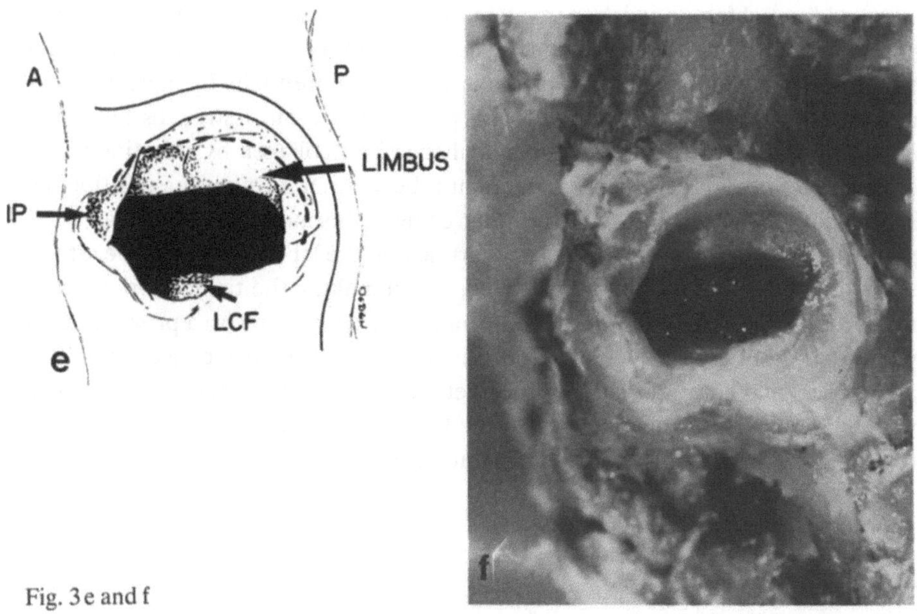

Fig. 3e and f

This case demonstrates that acetabular deformation may occur at an extremely early age. Nishimura felt that congenital deformities were rare among fetuses aborted prior to twenty weeks of gestation. The fetus described above was only slightly older and showed major structural changes affecting only one hip. Laurenson (1964) reported a comparable specimen from a 26-week-old fetus presumed to have arthrogryposis multiplex congenita. This specimen had bilateral dislocations with formation of false acetabula and beginning inversion of the acetabular margin. Of further interest was the observation that despite extensive soft tissue changes in the acetabulum, the development of the osseous portions of the ilium was relatively unaffected. The flatness of the acetabular roof occurs early in fetal development (Laurenson, 1965). Roentgenograms of other fetuses (even near term) with obvious acetabular changes did not always show obvious accompanying roentgenographic changes. The presence of a normal acetabular index should not be construed to mean that a hip is normal.

The acetabulum is a composite of all three portions of the pelvis – ilium, ischium and pubis – with the ischium forming the posteroinferior portion, the pubis the anteroinferior portion and the ilium the superior or acetabular roof. Iliac ossification usually begins by the eighth to ninth week and rapidly spreads throughout the cartilaginous *anlage* as the primary center. The apparent slope of this ossification center only indicates the extent to which the roof region has ossified, and does not represent the true shape of the cartilaginous acetabulum, whether normal or abnormal.

The finding of early hypertrophy of the hyaline-fibrocartilage margin of the labrum, despite obvious marginal eversion of the bulk of this structure, suggests that the hypertrophied limbus may develop by continued tissue remodeling, rather than abrupt inversion.

An additional factor which seems to play a role in susceptibility to CDH is the hormonal alteration accompanying the last trimester of pregnancy. Certain fetal tissues, such as the hip capsule, may be affected preferentially by maternal hormones, especially those concerned with pelvic relaxation. Estrogens block the maturation of newly synthesized tropocollagen into collagen by affecting cross-linkage (Henneman). If the proximal femur, because of intrauterine positioning, is already beginning to distend the joint capsule, hormonal changes may compound the rate of distension. The fibrocartilage of the labrum may also be affected, with abnormal cross-linkage of the collagen making the tissue more susceptible to deformation. Smith described a multigravid woman with a previous child with unilateral CDH in whom serial urinary estrogen (estrone, estradiol-17B, and estriol) and amniotic estriol levels were abnormally high; the child was born with bilateral CDH. Smith suggested the familial tendency of CDH may be the result of an inborn error of estrogen metabolism.

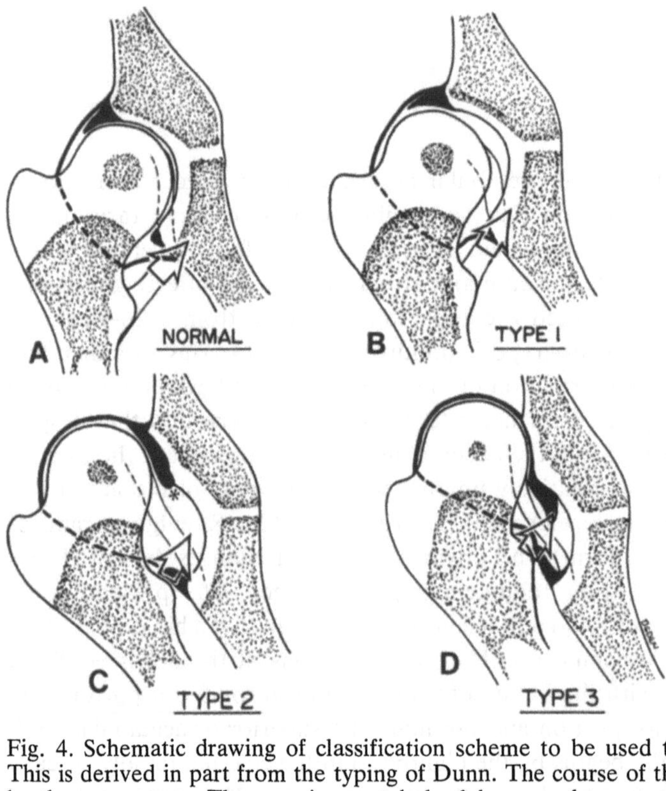

Fig. 4. Schematic drawing of classification scheme to be used throughout the article. This is derived in part from the typing of Dunn. The course of the iliopsoas is depicted by the *open arrow*. The superior acetabular labrum and transverse acetabular ligament are *blackened*. All hips are approximately 6 postnatal months. (a) – normal hip, with acetabular labrum enveloping femoral head. (b) – positionally unstable or subluxatable hip, with lateralization of femoral head and mild distortion (eversion) of acetabular labrum. (c) – subluxated hip, with significant eversion of labrum (and some marginal inversion – *asterisk*), and beginning inversion of transverse acetabular ligament by translocating iliopsoas. (d) – dislocated hip, with formation of false acetabulum against ilium, inversional hypertrophy of the labrum to form the limbus and inversion of inferior capsule and transverse acetabular ligament into the true acetabulum by the translocated iliopsoas

The Perinatal Period

The times of maximum susceptibility to hip subluxation and dislocation appear to be the last trimester and the neonatal period. Ralis and McKibbin have shown that the depth of the acetabulum and overall coverage of the femoral head gradually decrease to a minimum around full-term. The femoral head has a significant effect on the contour of the acetabulum, and may profoundly change the acetabular shape due to intrauterine position, thereby accentuating the normal process of decreasing acetabular depth. As will be shown, however, the depth changes so induced are eccentric, causing the acetabulum to change from a circular structure to an elliptical one. Dunn (1976b) performed a detailed study of neonatal hips and devised a classification scheme based primarily upon the shape of the acetabular margin, eversion or inversion of the limbus, and gross contour of the femoral head. The three types, as illustrated in Figure 4, represent positional instability or subluxability (type 1), subluxation (type 2), and dislocation (type 3). His scheme very adequately explains the spectrum of the disease, but minimizes or neglects other important factors, particularly the roles of femoral anteversion and intrauterine position, and the possibility that "inversion" of the limbus may not be as straightforward as usually conceived. But since his classification scheme is useful, it will be employed for the following case presentations:

Type 1: Several positionally unstable hips were found among stillborn fetuses. All had unilateral involvement. All had flexion and adduction contractures that were not easily corrected into an anatomic position even after all musculature was removed. The capsule very obviously appeared to be the major limiting factor to complete abduction and extension. The femoral heads did not exhibit any gross contour deformities other than anteversion, which ranged from 60° to 90°. In each case the obvious structural deformities involved the acetabulum (Fig. 5). All had mild, but variable, changes in the acetabular rim, involving both the hyaline and fibrocartilage components. Each acetabulum was shallow relative to the contralateral hip. Figure 5 demonstrates a minimally involved acetabulum with limited involvement of the anterior and superior walls and virtually no involvement of the posterior wall. Figure 5 b shows an example of anterior and posterior wall deficiency, with eversion and enlargement of the superior rim; this case also demonstrated minimal "inversion" of the fibrocartilage-hyaline cartilage junction posteriorly, despite eversion of the bulk of the fibrocartilaginous labrum. The last case (Fig. 5c) showed anterior deficiency with posterior eversion (again with a suggestion of marginal "inversion" at junction of articular surface and labrum). When the femora were placed in the acetabula, it became evident that the anteverted femoral head was exerting pressure on the deformed superior and posterior rims, while the anterior deformity appeared to be the result of pressure from the lesser trochanter and medial femoral metaphysis, as well as the femoral head. If the femur was placed in a position of flexion and moderate abduction (less than 60°), the head could be directed more centrally and appeared to exert less eccentric pressure on the superior and posterior rims. Furthermore, in this position the femoral metaphysis and lesser trochanter were no longer resting against the deficient anterior rim. Similar mild changes may exist in the slightly older child, and appear to be the cause of marginal osseous changes seen during roentgenography (Fig. 6).

These cases demonstrate the mild deformities along the acetabular margins, which lessen femoral head coverage and allow instability in certain positions. All cases had significant femoral anteversion. The apparent intrauterine positions were such that excessive pressure was directed against the anterior wall by the

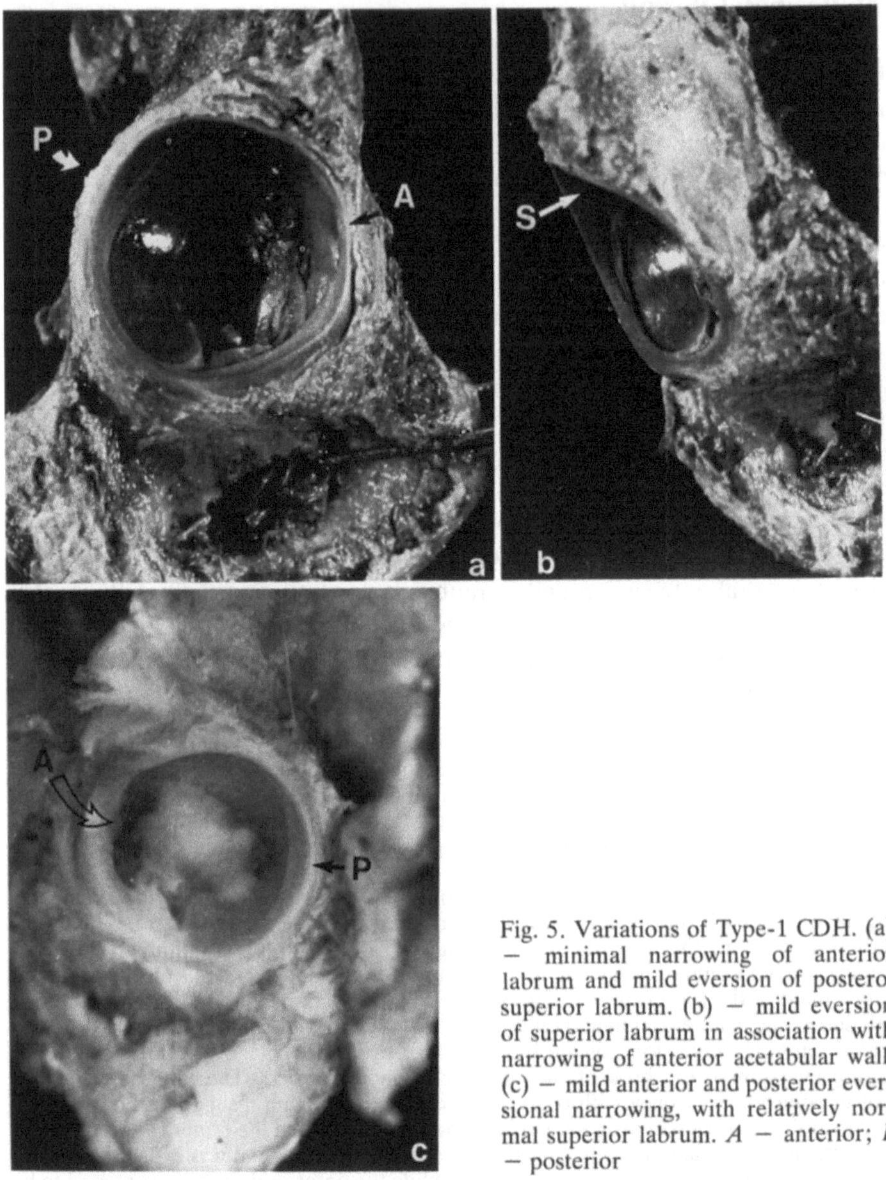

Fig. 5. Variations of Type-1 CDH. (a) – minimal narrowing of anterior labrum and mild eversion of posterosuperior labrum. (b) – mild eversion of superior labrum in association with narrowing of anterior acetabular wall. (c) – mild anterior and posterior eversional narrowing, with relatively normal superior labrum. *A* – anterior; *P* – posterior

lesser trochanter, iliopsoas tendon and femoral head and metaphysis, causing anterior marginal deficiency. The anteverted femoral head also placed excessive pressure on the superior and posterior margins, causing the fibrocartilaginous labrum to evert. However, while the majority of the posterosuperior labrum was everting, small portions of the fibrocartilage at the junction with articular hyaline cartilage were starting to hypertrophy and suggested early concomitant inversion of the inner portion of the labrum. This strongly suggests that inversion may not be an acute phenomenon, but rather a gradual tectonic change. Placement of the hips in a flexion-abduction position created better coverage of

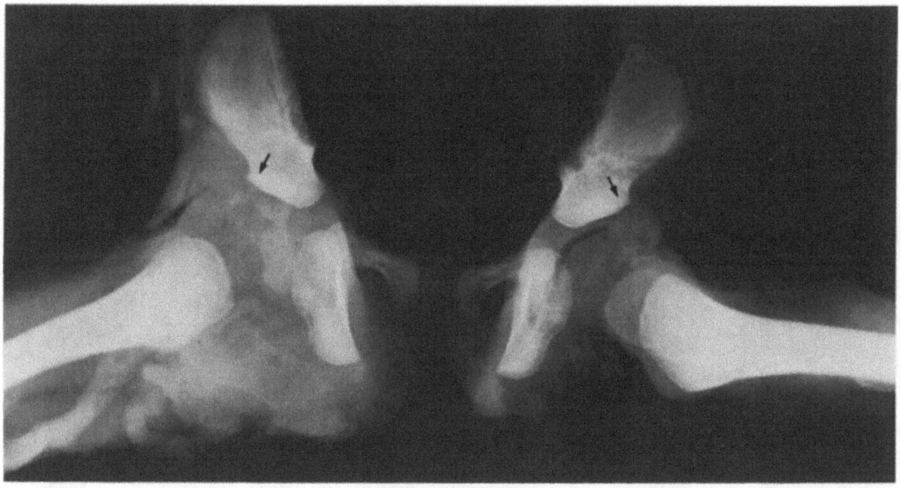

Fig. 6. Two-month-old infant with myelomeningocoele. The acetabulum showed minimal (Type-1) changes, but the roentgenogram showed increased deformity of the lateral portion of the osseous roof

the head and directed pressure centrally than eccentrically. This position particularly decreased potentially deforming contact along the anterior margin, and lessened contact superiorly and posteriorly. The tendency of the labrum to evert superiorly, the anterior deficiency and the increased pressure from the anteverted, subluxatable femoral head undoubtedly all contribute to the decreased ossification of the acetabular roof that manifests itself as an increase in the acetabular index (steepness or acclivity).

Type 2: The femoral heads again demonstrated significant anteversion, and were beginning to show loss of sphericity (Fig. 7a). The acetabula were more deformed, particularly showing increased eversion of the posterosuperior margin, which contributed, together with the anterior deficiency, to the shallow acetabula (Fig. 7b). Attempts to place the hips in various positions of treatment were not as successful due to increased incongruency between femoral head and acetabulum. The hips removed from an older child (three months postnatal) showed marked eversion of the posterosuperior rim on gross examination, and increased acclivity on roentgenography (Fig. 8a). On an air arthrogram of the hip joint the superior displacement and distended capsule became quite evident (Fig. 8b, c). Attempted reduction was not successful due to fibrofatty tissue in the acetabulum and flattening of the acetabulum that caused incongruency of the components.

The hips in this category demonstrated a gradual change manifested by femoral head deformity and eversion of the posterosuperior labrum. In type 1 the mildly deformed acetabulum was elliptical in shape. In type 2 eccentric eversion and hypertrophy made the marginal contours much more irregular. Reduction was less satisfactory than in type 1, but placement in usual treatment positions did lessen eccentric contact between femoral head and acetabulum.

Type 3: The most severe deformations of the acetabular margins were encountered in this group. Figure 9 shows roentgenographic findings of a child who expired several days after birth. It was impossible to accurately reduce this hip due to contractures of the capsule (all muscles had been removed). Following capsulotomy reduction was still un-

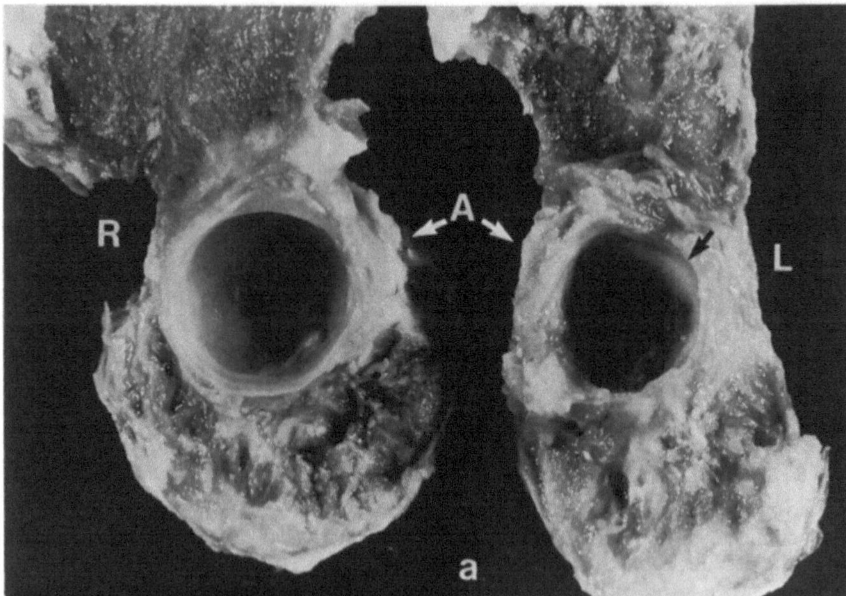

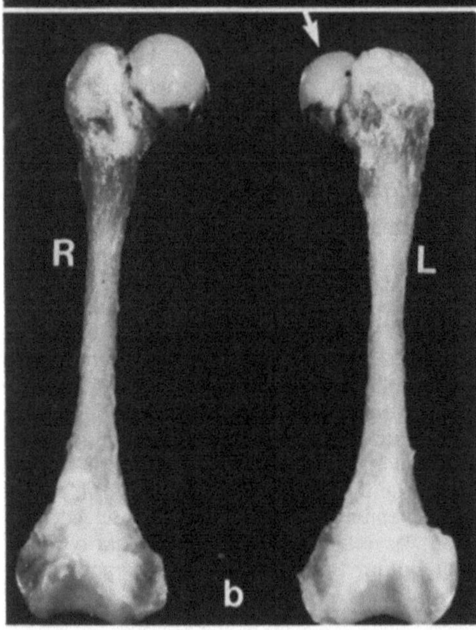

Fig. 7. Type-2 deformity in full-term stillborn. (a) – normal and deformed acetabula. (b) – normal and minimally deformed femora. The left acetabulum showed loss of the anterior (*A*) wall and eversion of the postero-superior labrum. The left proximal femur showed a mild "varus" deformity, with a negative articulo-trochanteric distance, compared to the normal right side

satisfactory due to loss of femoral head sphericity and extreme acetabular deformity. Other completely dislocated hips demonstrated that marginal changes of inversion really were a combination of (presumed) initial eversion followed by inversional hypertrophy,

---

Fig. 8. Roentgenography of bilateral Type-2 lesion in a 3-month-old child. (a) – the *black arrow* shows some mild lateral acclivity and sclerosis of the osseous acetabular roof. The *white arrow* depicts the capsule and femoral head. (b) – the introduction of air delineates the joint capsule (*c*). (C) – manipulation delineates the ligamentum capitum femoris (*L*). The right side, with similar deformity, has been reduced easily, although the capsule is redundant, and would easily allow the deformity to recur

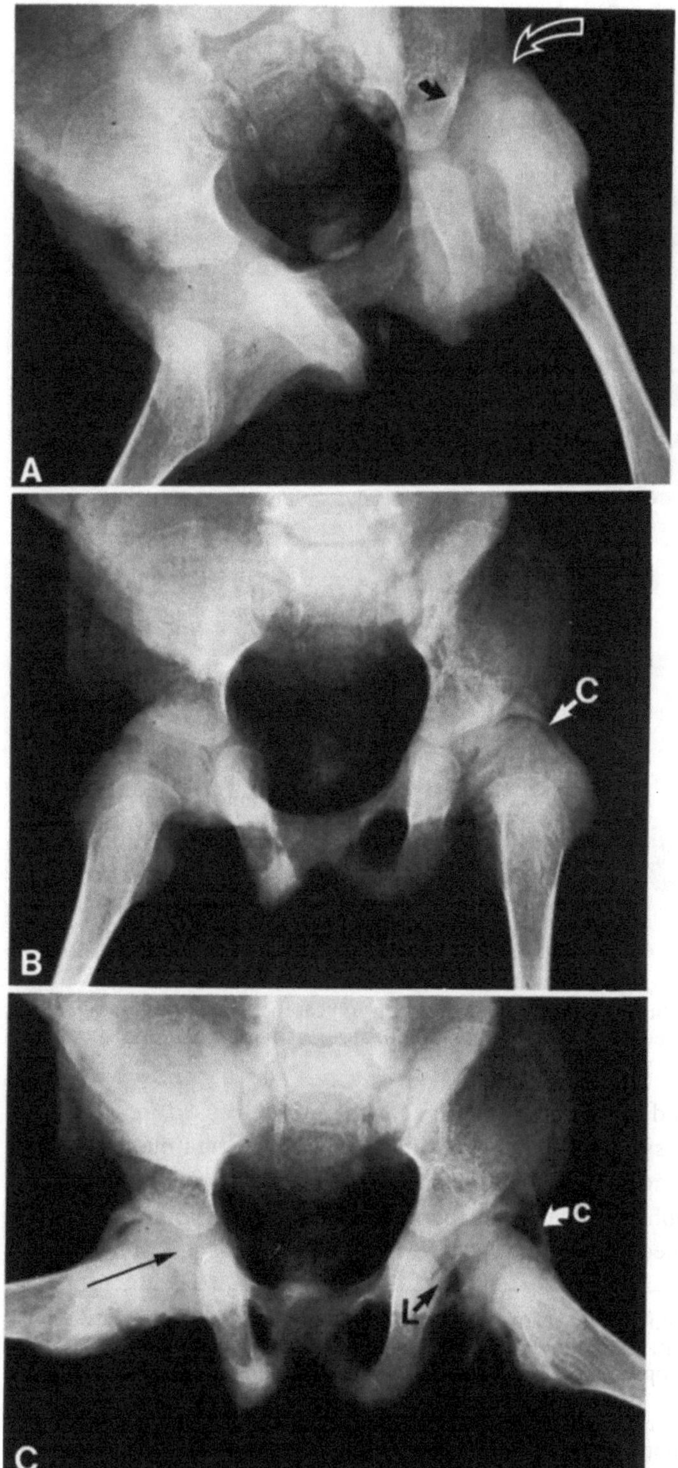

Fig. 8

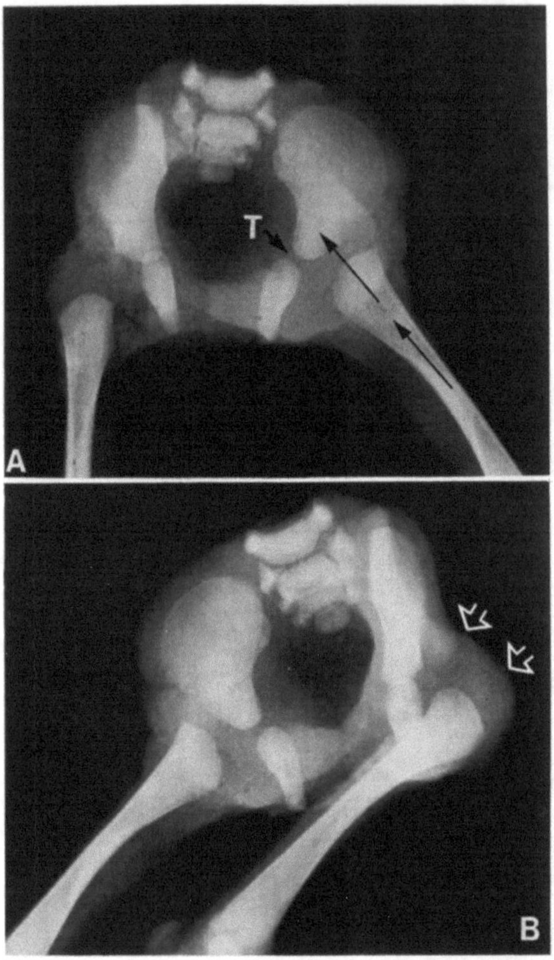

Fig. 9. Type-3 deformity. (a) – in the position easily assumed due to pathologic anatomic conformations the hip is obviously dislocated. *T* – triradiate cartilage. (b) – the proximal femur has been adducted to emphasize posterosuperior dislocation *(arrows)*

filling the vacated acetabulum (Fig. 10). The ligamentum capitis femoris was elongated in these cases and was pulled up from its normal origin, along with the transverse acetabular ligament.

These cases showed the most dramatic changes, which caused incongruency incompatible with easy reduction. However, placement in treatment positions suggested that rearrangement of joint reaction forces might possibly reverse the inversional hypertrophy. This suggests the possibility that excision of the limbus may not always be necessary. However, reversion of the changes may take an

---

Fig. 10. Type-3 deformity. *Top* – low-power photomicrograph to show relationships. *C* – capsule of hip joint; *LI* – limbus; *LCF* – ligamentum capitum femoris; *LT* – lesser trochanter; *IP* – iliopsoas (course shown by *arrows*). Middle-higher power showing capsule (*c*) attaching in normal position, eversion (*EV*) of more external portion of limbus, inversional hypertrophy (*INV*) of more internal portion of limbus, and fibrofatty (*F*) tissue between limbus and articular surface. *Bottom* – specimen stained to show fibrocartilaginous structure of limbus, with streaming of the tissue to accommodate pressure from the dislocated femoral head (histologic section provided by Dr. Aloysio Campos da Paz)

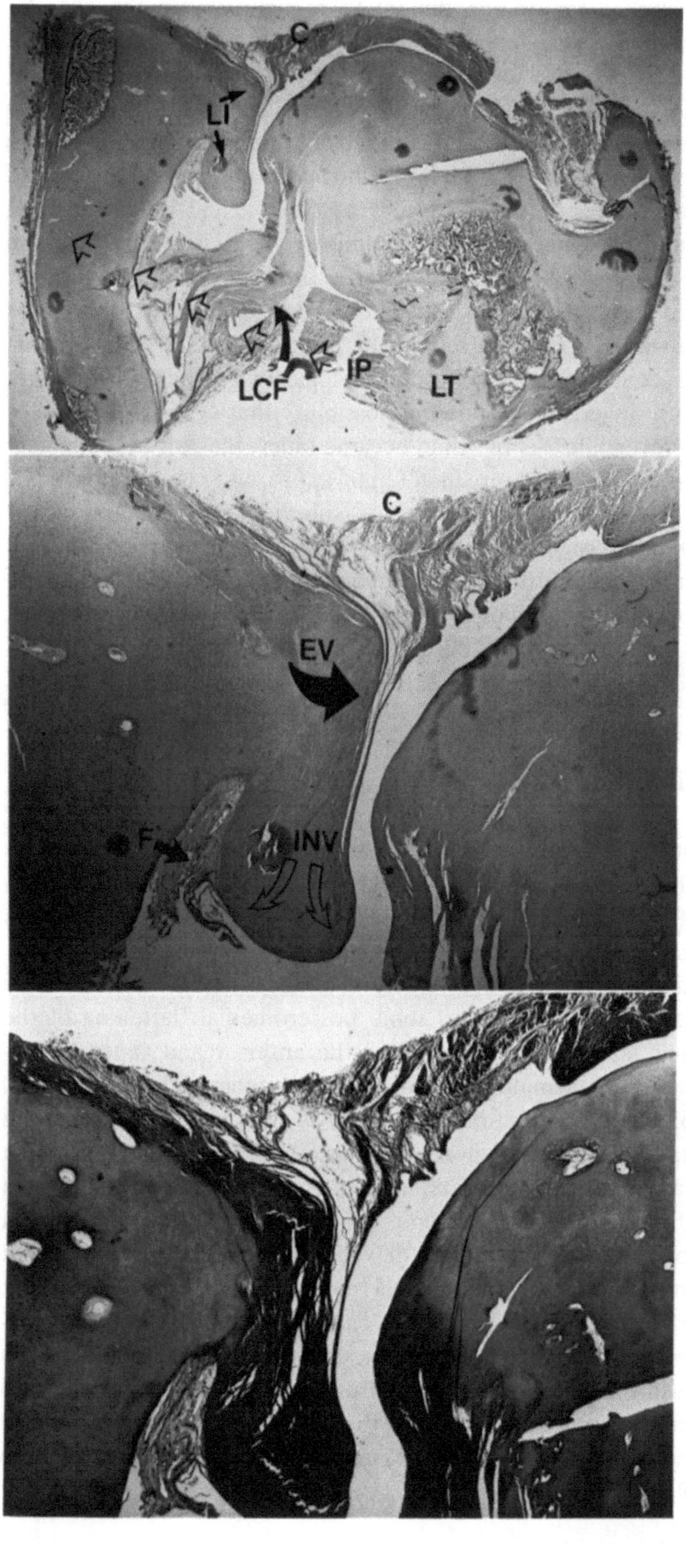

Fig. 10

exceedingly long time. A major impediment to reduction were the *capsular* contractures, rather than *muscular* contractures.

The changes in the perinatal period thus comprise a gradual spectrum of deformities involving both sides of the joint. These changes have been arbitrarily classified into three types. The subluxatable hip, by far the most common change encountered during newborn examination, showed minimum changes and adequate correction of the deforming forces by flexion and mild abduction treatment. The subluxated hip also showed improvement potential by these treatment positions, but femoral head changes were becoming evident. The most deformed hips were seen in the true dislocations. One of the most important structural changes was abnormal development of the limbus. However, this seemed to be a consequence of "flow" of the biologically plastic fibrocartilage, rather than an abrupt inversion, raising the possibility that even these changes might be gradually reversible. As the child became older, the pull of the gluteal musculature against the adducted proximal femur appeared to be a major factor accentuating the posterior (and to some degree, superior) deformity. In fact, if the hip, with its attendant capsular contractures, was brought toward extension, the proximal femur tended to piston posterosuperiorly out of the acetabulum, no matter if we were dealing with types 1, 2 or 3. Finally, there was *no* correlation between typical or teratologic hip and severity of anatomic changes.

Infancy and Childhood

Many orthopaedists have expressed the opinion that treatment of subluxations or dislocations of hip joints become increasingly difficult after the first three to four months of life, as cartilaginous deformation and soft tissue contractures supervene. Of those hips available for detailed pathological study, none from the perinatal period demonstrated *major* structural deformities. There definitely was mild to moderate anteversion and some posteromedial flattening of the proximal femur, and marginal changes along the anterior and superior acetabular rims, but these abnormalities did not always appear to be irreversible, even in the teratologic hips. The first year of life is characterized by a rate in growth that gradually decreases until a static rate is attained. This equilibrium rate will be maintained for several years, until the child enters the first growth spurt during the four to seven year range. While the prenatal and perinatal periods were associated with rapid growth which can result in femoral and acetabular deformities, the slower postnatal period growth rates imply that structural changes will occur more gradually. This would apply both to the progression of deformity in the unrecognized or untreated CDH as well as the gradual correction in the child treated by nonsurgical measures. While surgical methods are directed at acute correction of the deformity, it must be realized that nonsurgical methods (cast, splint, brace) may take many months or years to manifest acceptable and significant changes.

Available pathologic material from the period of infancy and childhood is extremely rare. Milgram and Tachdjian described a hip removed at autopsy from a 10-month-old child. The femur was anterosuperiorly displaced into a false acetabulum. Anteversion was only 20°. Despite the chronicity of dislocation, the proximal femur was only mildly deformed, while the acetabulum was much more adversely affected. The appearance of the limbus suggested gradual ingrowth rather than abrupt inversion. A comparable case from a 15-month-old female showed similar mild to moderate deformities:

Because of multiple recurrent medical problems (pneumonitis) this child had never been treated for a bilateral dislocation present from birth (Fig. 11). The correlative gross and roentgenographic findings of the right hip have been described previously (Ogden

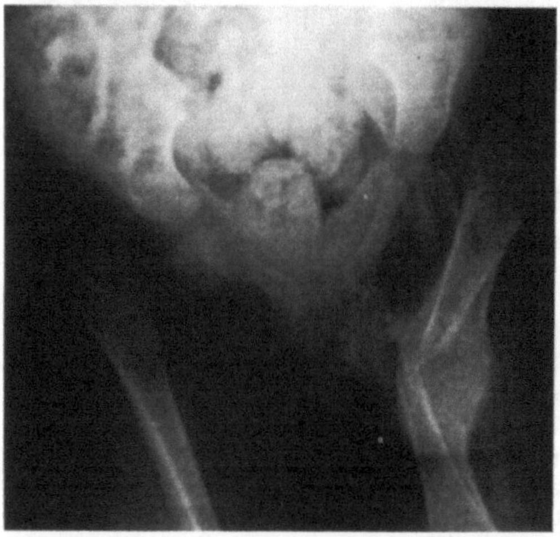

Fig. 11. Roentgenogram of 5-month-old infant with bilateral CDH and healed fracture of left femur. It is impossible to describe the exact pathologic anatomy in such a film (see Figs. 12–15)

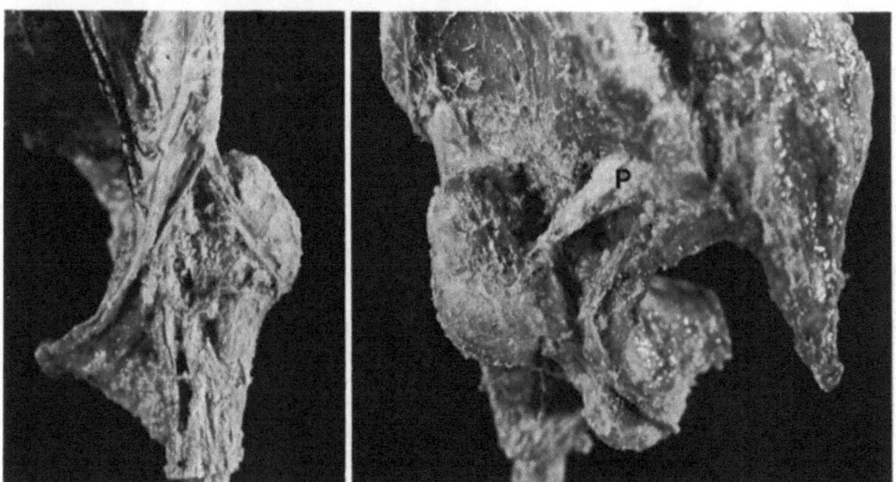

Fig. 12. Right – anterior view showing superior and lateral displacement. Left – posterior view of same hip. The piriformis (*P*) tendon was displaced and significantly contracted. Contracture of this tendon may be a problem overlooked in the difficult reduction

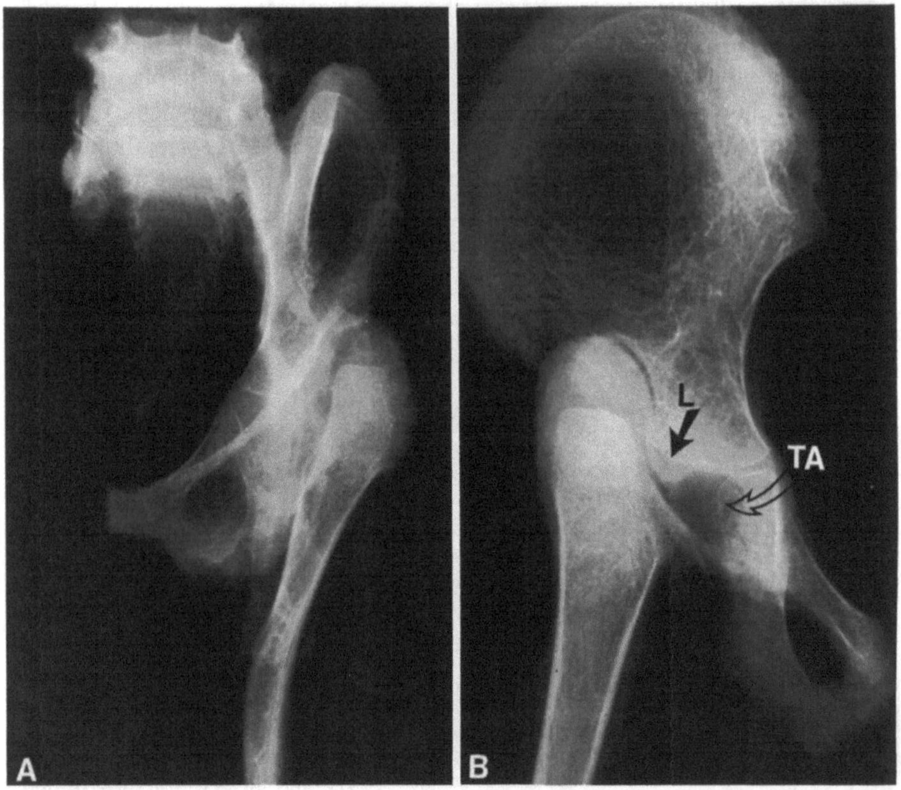

Fig. 13. Roentgenography of hip dislocation in 5-month-old female with arthrogryposis. (a) – dislocation of proximal femur against iliac wing, with lesser trochanter adjacent to true acetabulum. (b) – after introduction of air the false acetabulum is outlined, along with the apparently inverted limbus and true acetabulum

and Jensen). The right and left hips were almost comparable in degree of dislocation and structural changes. Gross examination (Fig. 12) of the left hip revealed an anterosuperior displacement and marked anteversion (70°; however, the femur had been fractured 10 months prior to death). The capsule was contracted anteriorly and distended posteriorly. The iliopsoas tendon crossed the true acetabulum to reach the lesser trochanter, causing a significant indentation of the attenuated, contracted inferior capsule. Posteriorly the most significant change appeared to be contracture of the piriformis tendon. Roentgenography showed an obvious dislocation (Fig. 13a); the soft tissue technique shows the outline of the laterally displaced femoral head. Air was injected into the capsule to outline the joint (Fig. 13b). This very readily demonstrated apparent inversion of the acetabular margin. The hips were then disarticulated (Fig. 14). The proximal femora were mildly deformed, but still retained most of their sphericity. Flattening was evident along the posterior portion of the femoral head. Both femora had significant valgus and anteversion. The true acetabulum initially appeared inadequate to accommodate the femoral head in any position of reduction, but once the reactive soft tissue was removed from the femoral head, there was more acetabular depth and a reasonable, although imperfect, reduction was possible. An obvious false acetabulum was in continuity with the true acetabulum. This appeared to result from a gradual, progressive, cranial displacement of the femur, with the capsule and labrum being pushed against the ilium and causing secondary osseous remodeling (increased acetabular index). Some of the most informative views were obtained by removing parts of the femur and pelvis to show chondroosseous relationships (Fig. 15). The acetabular margin (labrum) was primarily everted, but there were regions where hypertrophic ingrowth was occurring. These areas of ingrowth could easily be described as an inverted labrum, or limbus, especially on roentgenography.

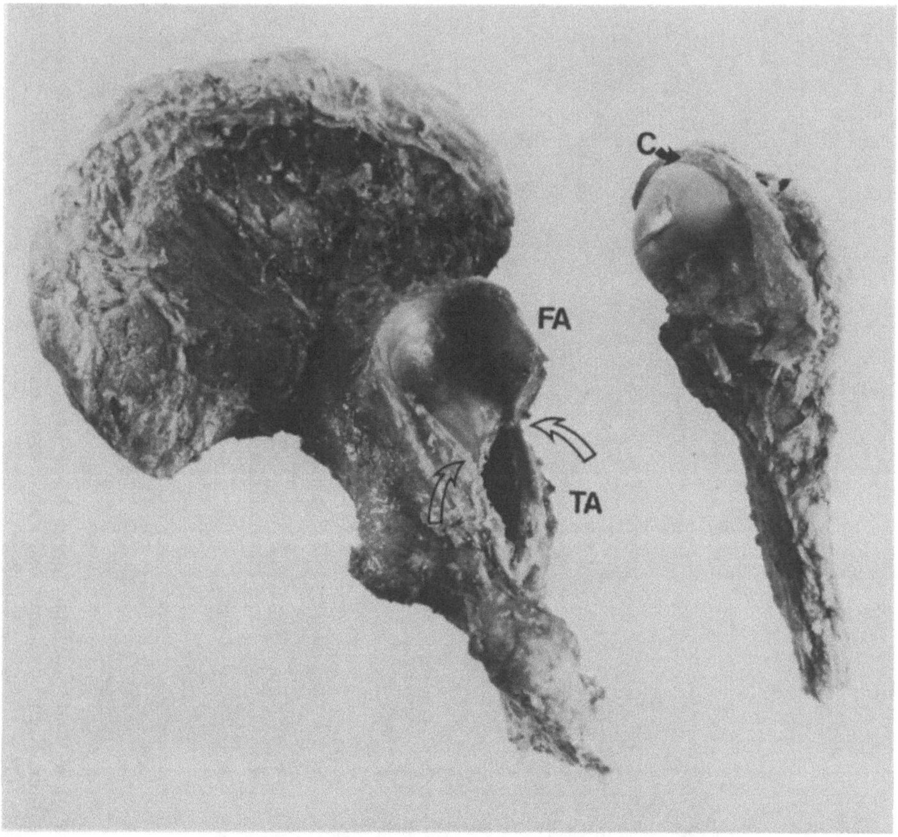

Fig. 14. Disarticulated right hip showing false acetabulum *(FA)* and true acetabulum *(TA)*. The *arrows* depict the "hour-glass" constriction of the region between the acetabula caused by the translocated iliopsoas tendon. The joint capsule *(C)* was adherent to the femoral head

Thus, despite 15 postnatal months of dislocation, and an unknown time period of changes in utero, both hips showed only moderate changes which probably could have been reversed with appropriate treatment. In the flexed, abducted position shown in figure 15, the femoral head was reasonably covered. These hips were unusual in the degree of symmetry of deformity. In general, one side is more involved than the other in bilateral cases.

The hips from two older children, in the 7–11 year range, were studied. Both children had gone through the first major growth spurt and showed very significant deformities of both the acetabulum and proximal femur that would have an adverse affect on any treatment modality.

The first specimen was removed from a seven year old child with a myelomeningocele. The gross specimen showed a posterosuperior dislocation (Fig. 16a), with a flexion contracture. The adductors did not have a significant contracture (in fact, the position of the hip was in mild abduction). The hip capsule was attenuated in the direction of dislocation (superiorly and posteriorly) and was contracted anteriorly and inferiorly. The lesser trochanter abutted against the superior portion of the pubic ramus and caused a marked indentation of the bone anterior to the true acetabulum, accentuating the

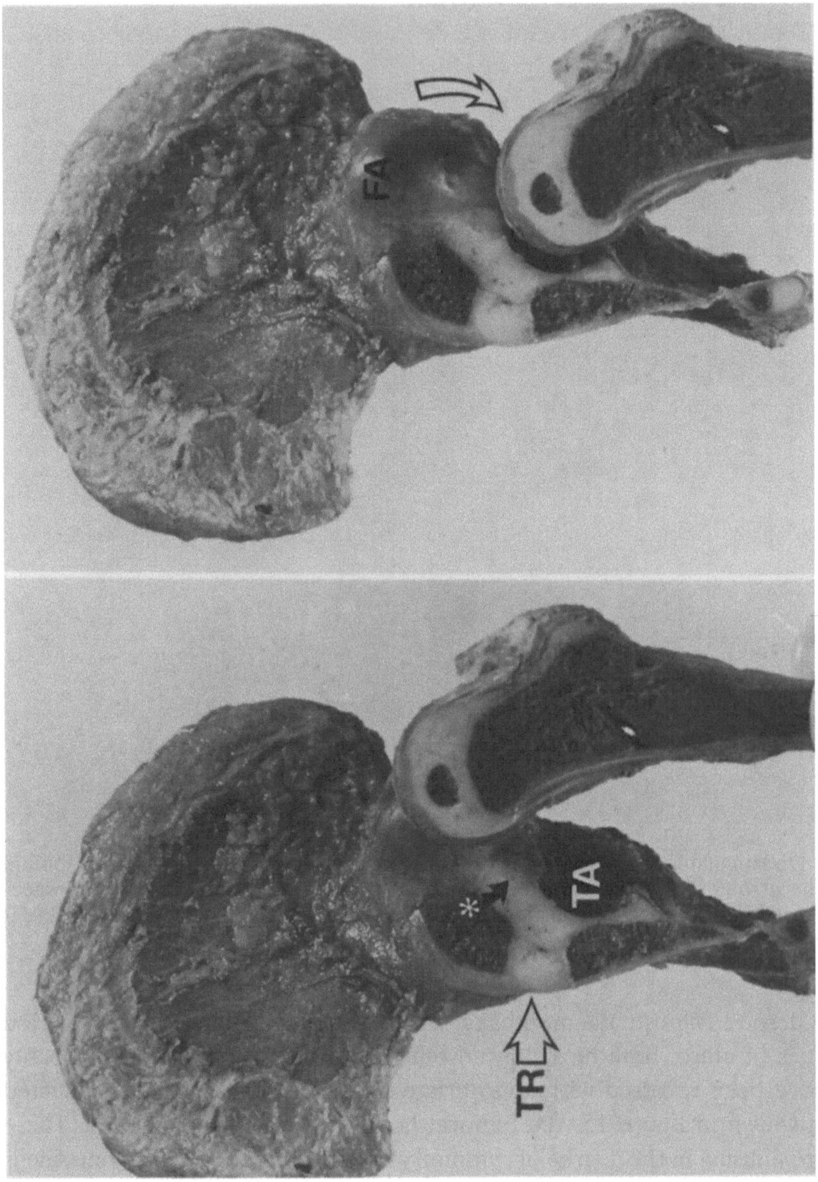

Fig. 15. Portions of the acetabulum and proximal femur have been removed to show chondroosseous relationships in a Type-3 dislocation. Right – femur dislocated into false acetabulum (*FA*). Left – femur reduced into true acetabulum (*TA*). *TR* – triradiate cartilage

anterior deficiency of this structure (Fig. 16b). The proximal femur had more than 110° of anteversion, as well as marked valgus (over 180° in the true AP plane). The lesser trochanter, in response to the tightness of the iliopsoas, was overgrown and much more prominent than in a normal femur (Fig. 16c). The femoral head was deformed in all areas and had lost its sphericity (Fig. 17a). The chronic pressure from the ligamentum capitis femoris (teres) had eroded away all articular cartilage in the medial region of the head of the femur. The acetabular labrum was variably deformed (Fig. 17b). There were obvious areas of eversion, and other areas, especially posterior, were suggestive of inversion. The irregularity of the margin between the true and false acetabulum had obviously contributed to the deformity of the femoral head. Roentgenography showed a shallow true acetabulum and a well-formed false acetabulum (Fig. 18). The medial circumflex

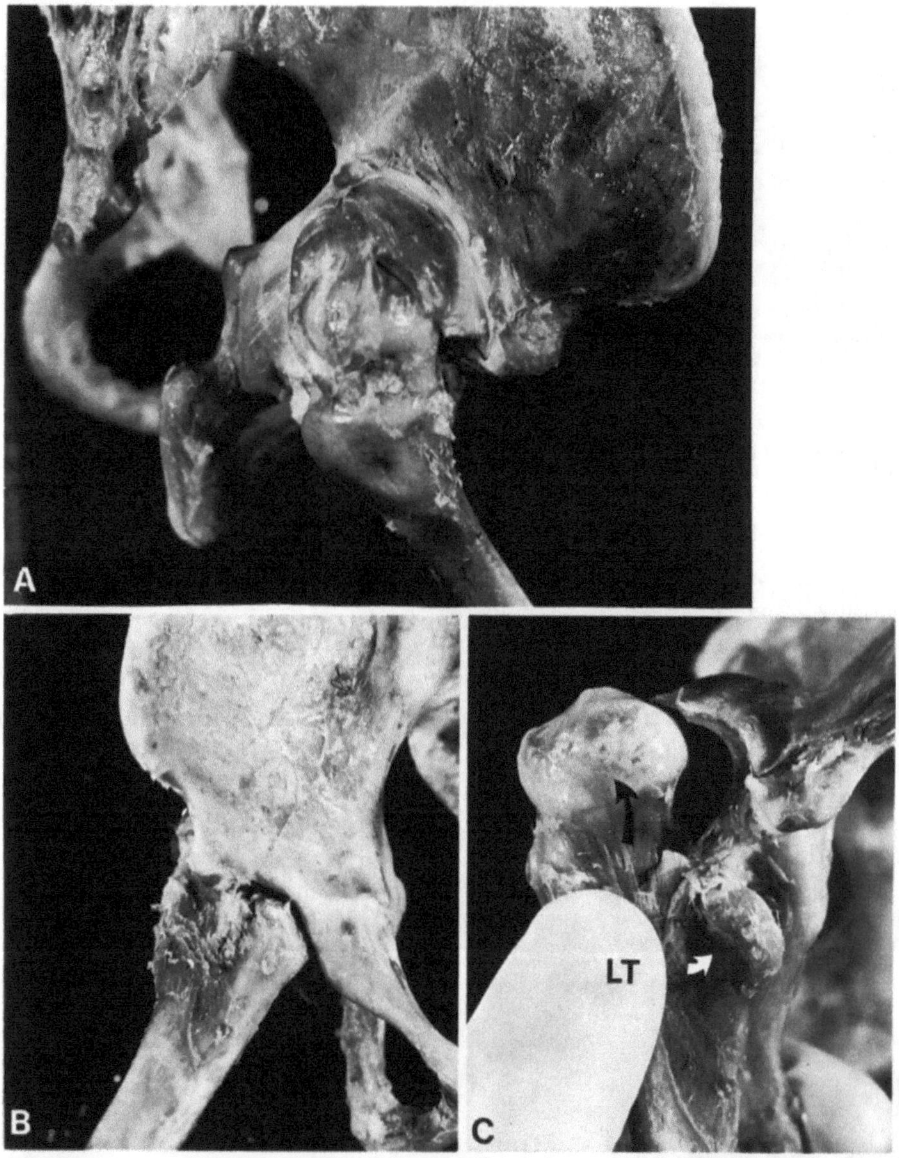

Fig. 16. (a) – posterosuperior dislocation of the right hip. (b) – anterior view, showing interlocking relationship of lesser trochanter and pubic ramus. (c) – overgrowth of lesser trochanter *(LT)* and severe valgus deformity of femoral head

artery had shifted concomitant with the iliopsoas, and coursed between the iliopsoas tendon and the pubic ramus. The capsule indented into the true acetabulum. This area had a moderate amount of reactive tissue that made isolation of the artery difficult.

This specimen demonstrated several significant features that may be seen in the older child, irrespective of the hip being considered a typical or teratologic dislocation. First, there was a positional shift of the artery which would render it more susceptible to occlusion or transection. The cephalad shift of the proximal

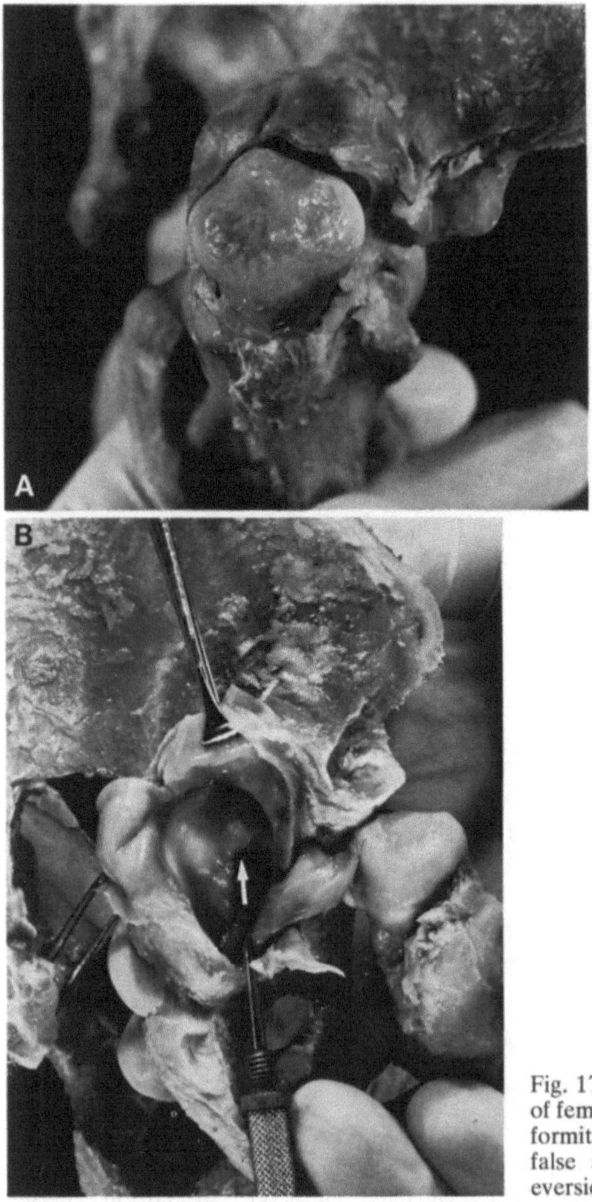

Fig. 17. (a) – deformity of contour of femoral head. (b) – irregular deformity of margin between true and false acetabula, showing areas of eversion and inversion

femur brought the lesser trochanter closer to the pubic ramus, and the iliopsoas tendon had a longer course over bone, both factors increasing the risk of vascular compromise. The femur was twisted into extreme anteversion (beyond 90°) and valgus (beyond 180°). These deformities obviously occurred over an extended period of time in response to biologic plasticity. The lesser trochanter showed deformed overgrowth that only compounded the deformity. The femoral head had become grossly deformed, while the acetabulum was less involved, except for the irregular marginal deformity. The primary acetabular deformity appeared to be lack of normal depth.

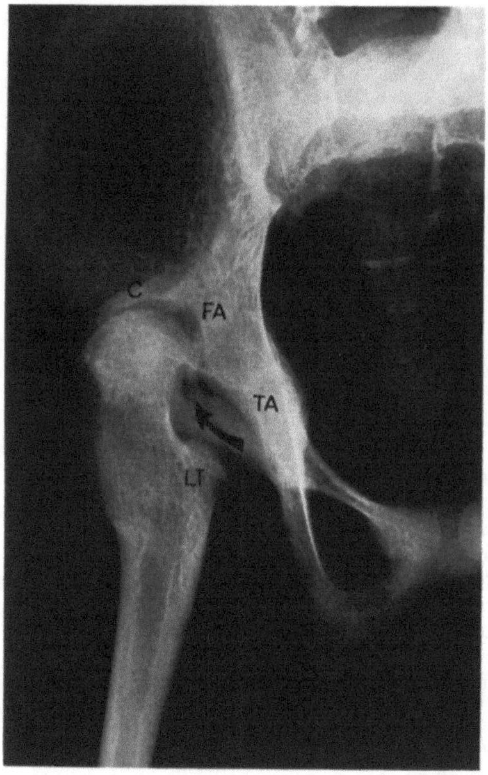

Fig. 18. Roentgenogram of dislocation in the older child, showing capsule *(C)*, false acetabulum *(FA)*, true acetabulum *(TA)*, and lesser trochanter *(LT)*. The *arrow* depicts the ligamentum capitum femoris coming out of the true acetabulum

The second specimen was removed from an 11-year-old child without known musculoskeletal pathology. The proximal femur was dislocated superiorly and slightly anteriorly, and had approximately a 30° flexion and 10° adduction contracture (Fig. 19). The iliopsoas tendon crossed the true acetabulum and depressed the inferior capsule into the acetabulum (Fig. 19). The transverse acetabular ligament was hypertrophied and

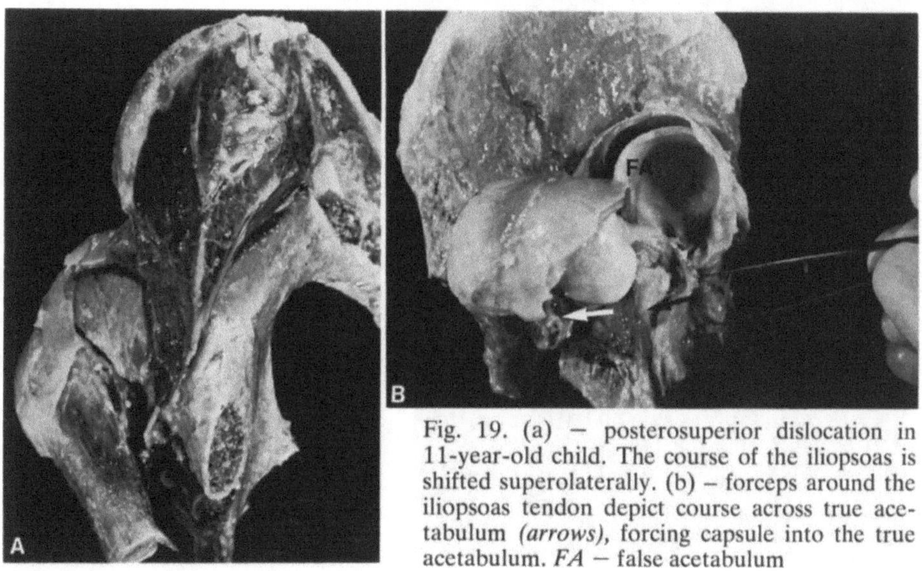

Fig. 19. (a) – posterosuperior dislocation in 11-year-old child. The course of the iliopsoas is shifted superolaterally. (b) – forceps around the iliopsoas tendon depict course across true acetabulum *(arrows)*, forcing capsule into the true acetabulum. *FA* – false acetabulum

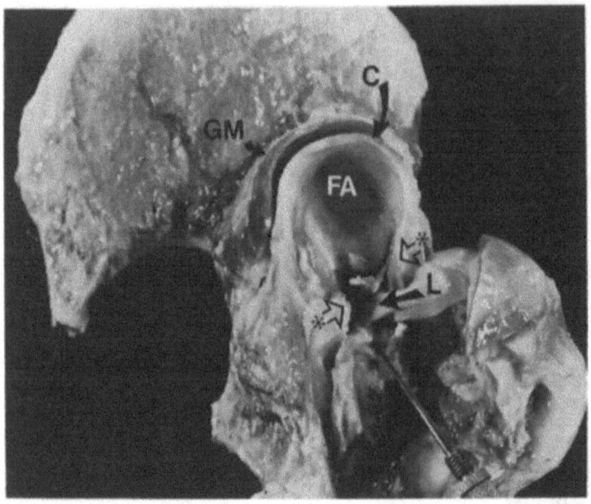

Fig. 20. Disarticulated specimen showing gluteus minimus *(GM)* and capsule *(C)* above false acetabulum *(FA)*. The ligamentum capitum femoris *(L)* can be followed into the true acetabulum (arrow). Open arrows and *asterisks* show "hour-glass" capsular indentation at junction of true and false acetabula

displaced into the acetabulum. The ligamentum capitis femoris (teres) was elongated and could be followed from the false acetabulum into the true acetabulum (Fig. 20). The medial circumflex artery was displaced superiorly along with the iliopsoas and was in close proximity to the pubic ramus. Further, the course of the posteroinferior branch of the artery between the iliopsoas and inferior femoral neck would appear to make the vessel extremely susceptible to temporary occlusion. The femoral head was not as severely deformed as the previous teratologic case, but there certainly was moderate posterior flattening and 80° of anteversion (in contrast, the opposite hip was not displaced, but showed increased anteversion of ninety degrees, valgus, and a shallow

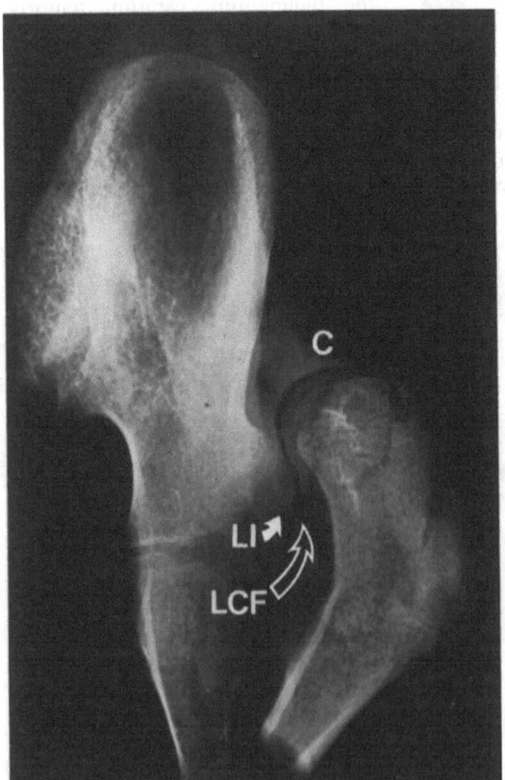

Fig. 21. Roentgenogram of specimen from 11-year-old child, showing capsule *(C)*, hypertrophic inversion of limbus *(LI)*, and ligamentum capitum femoris *(LCF)* coming from true acetabulum

acetabulum with anterior marginal deficiency). Roentgenography demonstrated the true acetabulum with irregular ossification in the roof, a false acetabulum with increased soft tissue between the capsule and ilium, and femoral valgus and moderate deformation of the femoral ossification center (Fig. 21).

This specimen proved to be less deformed than the previous example, corroborating the observation that a teratologic hip is more severely involved. However, the basic changes were comparable, and certainly would have made reduction and construction of an acetabular roof difficult.

Subluxation in Infancy and Childhood

The antecedent case presentations and discussions have focused upon the concept that intrauterine and perinatal factors may predispose the hip to

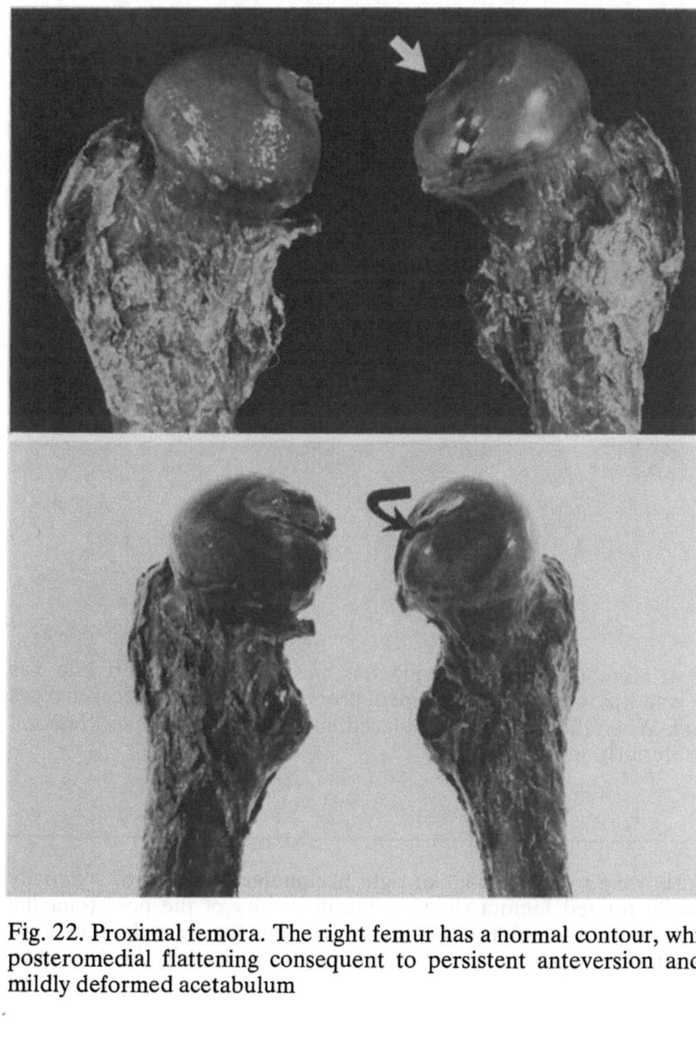

Fig. 22. Proximal femora. The right femur has a normal contour, while the left femur has posteromedial flattening consequent to persistent anteversion and pressure against a mildly deformed acetabulum

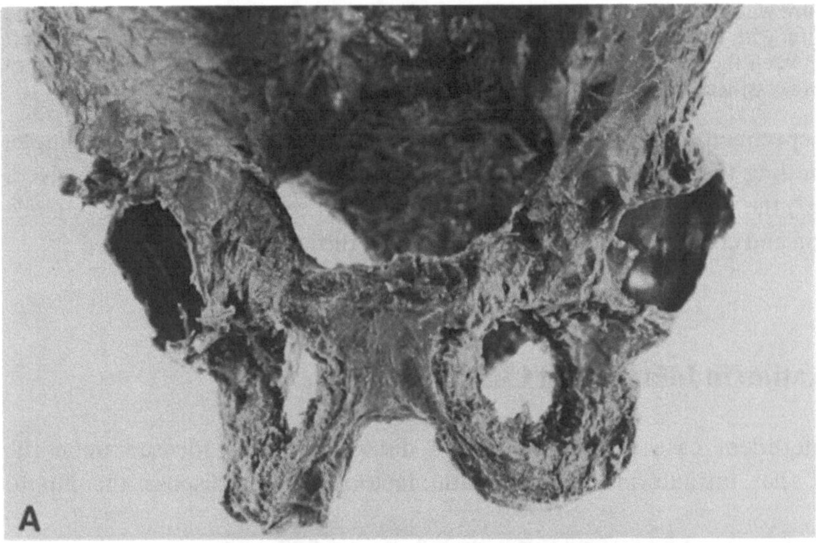

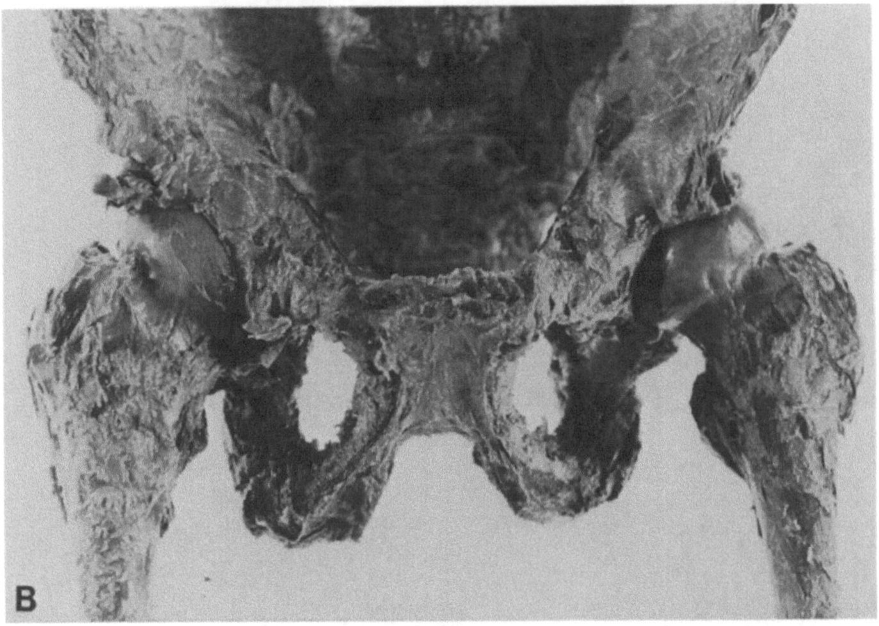

Fig. 23. Appearance of acetabula. The right side was normal, while the left side was shallow. The anterior wall was narrow and deformed, probably due to reciprocal changes from the femoral head. When the femora were placed in the acetabula the left femoral head was uncovered anteriorly and superiorly

---

Fig. 24. (a) – pelvis showing round contour of right acetabulum and loss of sphericity of left. (b) – externally rotated femora showing the deformity of the posteromedial left femur. (c) – maximum internal rotation shows congruency on right, but poor relationship on left. The arrow points to an area of increased acclivity in the lateral osseous acetabular roof

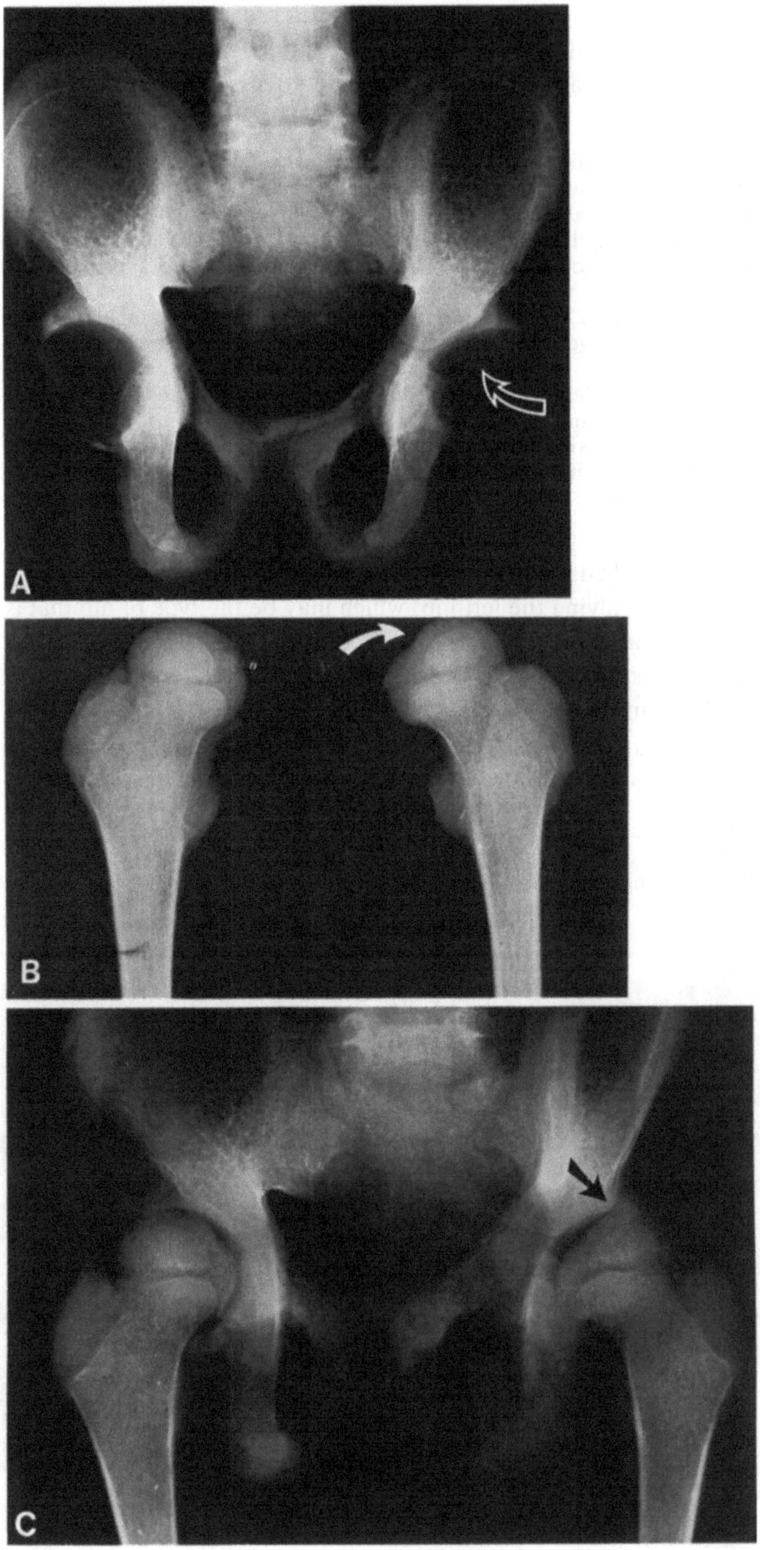

Fig. 24

progressive dislocation. However, it is conceivable that some hips so affected during early development will not progress to dislocation, but may retain some deformity and be classified as subluxation. Two examples of subluxation were found in the current study:

The first set of hips were obtained from a 2-year-old female. The right hip was normal, although the proximal femur was slightly anteverted (50°). The left hip had several structural differences. The acetabulum was more shallow than on the right side and had a very narrow anterior wall, as well as thinning of the superior labrum. The acetabulum was slightly ovoid in a superoinferior direction. The proximal femur showed approximately 70–80° of anteversion. There was a significant posteromedial flattening and indentation of the femoral head (Fig. 22). When the femur was placed in the acetabulum there was an obvious lack of coverage anteriorly when compared to the other side (Fig. 23). Roentgenograms showed that there were structural deformities in the osseous and cartilaginous elements of the left hip, but not the right. However, despite the obvious gross changes, the acetabular indices appeared relatively normal, with just a slight marginal eversion of the osseous roof on the left side (Fig. 24). When the gross specimen was manipulated to duplicate the innominate osteotomy of Salter, the femoral head was covered much more adequately. However, when then assuming weight-bearing positions the proximal femur was not covered as well.

This case very succinctly demonstrates a mild, unilateral deformity with many CDH characteristics (involving the left hip) which may be the type of hip that is predisposed to later arthritic changes, even though a significant superior displacement did not occur. Complete correction would have required surgery on both sides of the joint.

The second set of hips was obtained from a 5-year-old child. Both acetabula were shallow and elongated in a superior/inferior direction. The superior labrum was also thin and mildly hypertrophic. The anterior wall of the acetabulum was deficient in both labrum and hyaline/articular cartilage (Fig. 25). The function of the anterior wall had been replaced by a markedly attenuated, elongated anterior capsule (Fig. 25). Both femoral heads had seemingly normal sphericity when viewed anteriorly but very evident

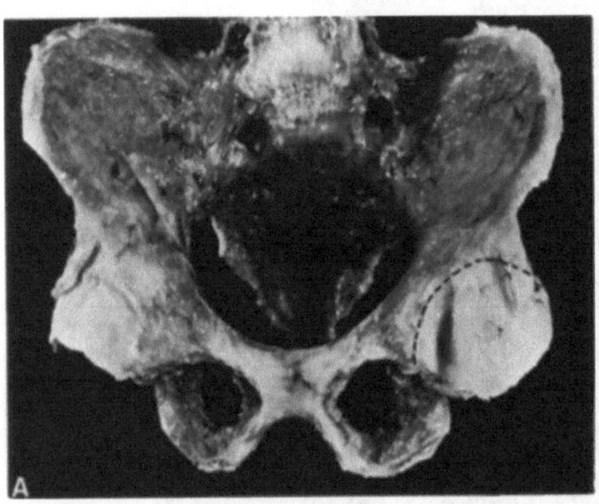

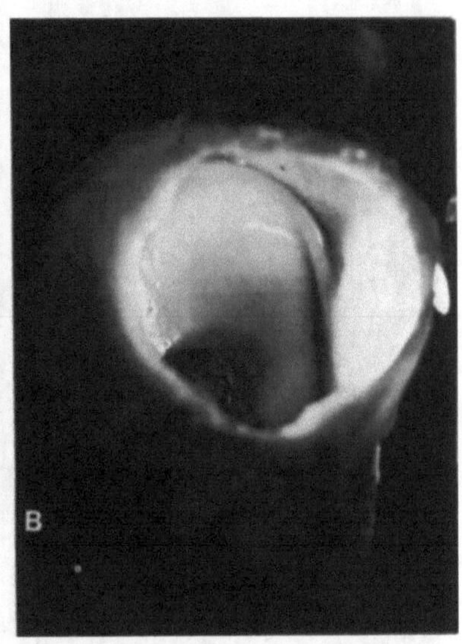

Fig. 25. (a) – pelvis, showing extensive anterior capsule. Extent of anterior acetabular rim is indicated by the *broken line.* (b) – transilluminated view of shallow right acetabulum showing superior/inferior elongation and minimal anterior wall

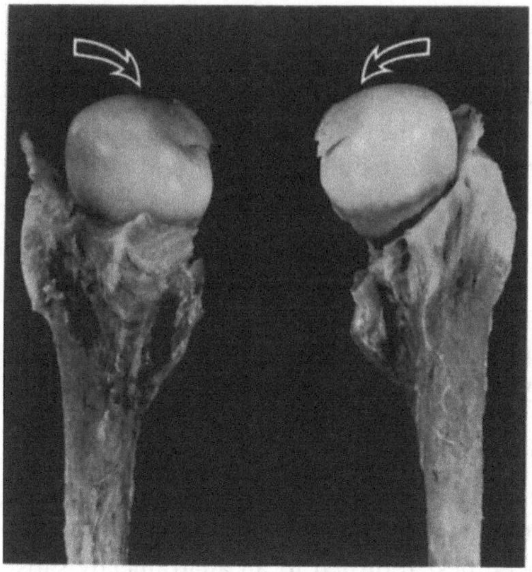

Fig. 26. Anterior, externally rotated view of femora to show the posteromedial flattening

posterosuperior flattening when viewed from behind, although the deformities were not symmetric (Fig. 26). There was approximately seventy degrees of anteversion bilaterally. Roentgenography showed a relatively normal appearance of the right acetabulum, while the left showed some marginal inclination (Fig. 27). If the proximal femora were placed in marked internal rotation they had a seemingly normal contour of the femoral head; however, if externally rotated, the superoposterior flattening became evident. Placement of both hips in the "Salter" position showed improved coverage, but attempts to subsequently place the femora in ambulatory position showed again that the uncorrected anteversion caused poor coverage of the femoral head, although not as severe as in the previous case.

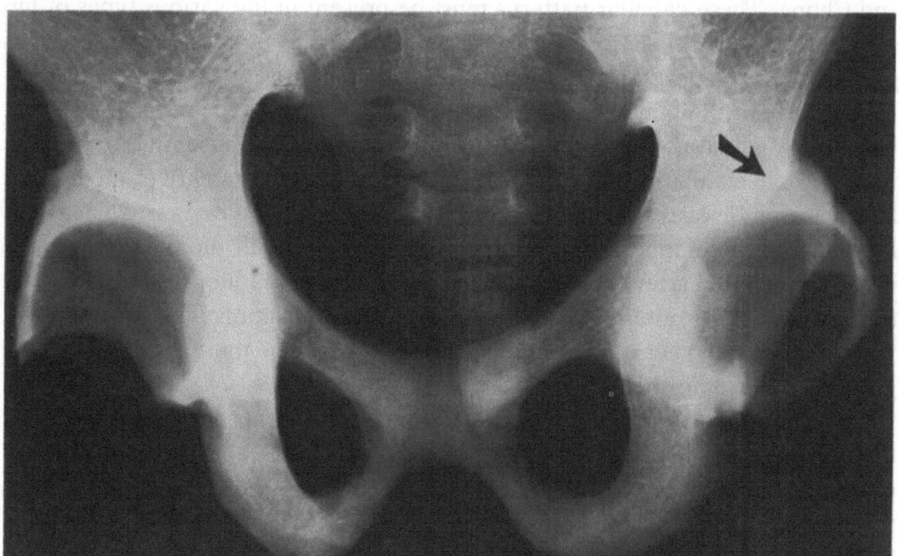

Fig. 27. Roentgenography of the pelvis. The acetabular acclivities were within normal limits. The only significant finding was the lateral angulation of the osseous roof *(arrow)*, also seen in other cases of subluxation (both in the perinatal and childhood periods)

These cases both illustrate mild acetabular dysplasia that included supero-inferior elongation, anterior wall deficiency and mild eversion of the superior hyaline component, in conjunction with an anteverted, deformed femoral head. In the apparent functional resting position the femoral head was uncovered anteriorly and the areas of deformity of the acetabulum and femoral head were the areas of chronic contact that had become deformed consequent to biologic plasticity. Why these hips, which had all the early findings presumed to predispose to eventual dislocation, did not dislocate, is not certain. These chronically subluxated hips may represent the long-term consequences of the type 1 hip dysplasia, which is an intrinsically unstable hip in the perinatal period, but usually stabilizes rapidly, simply with abduction treatment (although ante-version generally persists).

Attempts to duplicate the Salter innominate osteotomy showed good coverage of the anterior femoral head. But when pelvis and femur were placed in a functional position, there was still a tendency to anterior subluxation. Each of these subluxations would have been best returned to an anatomically satisfactory position only by femoral *and* pelvic osteotomies.

The Blood Supply and Avascular Necrosis

The changing patterns of gross and microscopic circulation of the proximal femur during growth have been described recently in detail by Ogden (1974a) and Chung. These vascular patterns must be present in the various types of hip subluxation and dislocation, if one accepts the concept that this disorder is primarily one of progressive deformation rather than a true malformation (in which case concomitant vascular anomalies might also be expected). Since CDH is primarily an alteration of initially normal anatomy, the essential problem in regard to the circulation appears to be an increased susceptibility of medial and lateral circumflex vessels to damage or occlusion at several extraarticular areas. Particularly, there appears to be increased vulnerability at the point where the medial circumflex artery courses around the translocated iliopsoas tendon, and along the posterior intertrochanteric groove, where positional constraints (e.g., frog leg hip spica) may cause undue pressure between the vessels within the groove and the deformed acetabular rim.

The blood supply of the proximal femur stems primarily from the deep femoral artery, which gives off two significant branches – the lateral and medial circumflex arteries (Fig. 28). While the lateral circumflex artery invariably arises from the deep femoral artery, the medial circumflex artery may arise either from the deep femoral artery or as an independent vessel from the main femoral artery. The origin of these two vessels is usually at the level of the tendinous portion of the iliopsoas muscle, although the vessels are separated from this tendon by a fibrous sheath (Ogden, 1974b).

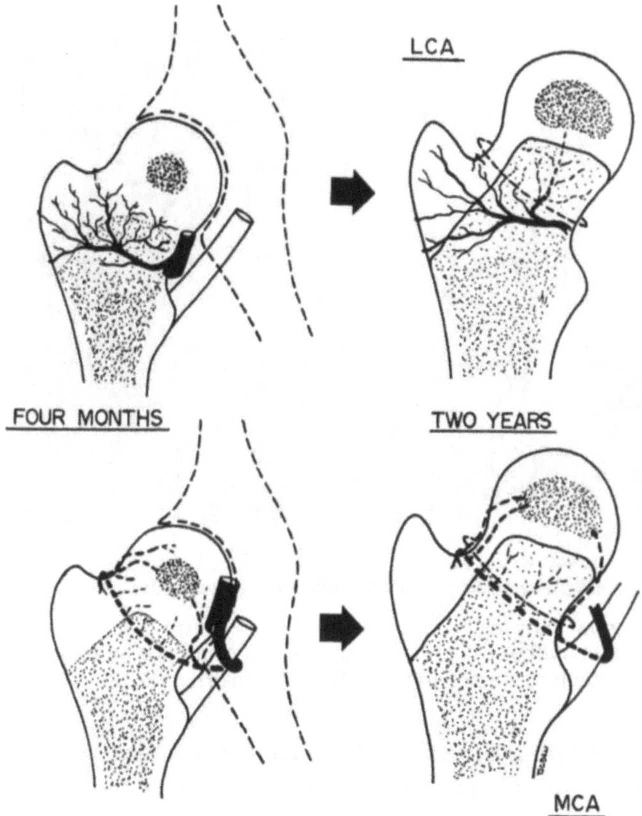

Fig. 28. Schematic representation of the circulatory patterns of the lateral *(LCA)* and medial *(MCA)* circumflex arteries at 4 months and 2 years. Most of the capital femoral ossification center and physis depends on the blood supply from the medial circumflex artery, which sends branches along the posteroinferior and posterosuperior femoral neck after wrapping around the iliopsoas tendon

The lateral circumflex artery crosses the lateral portion of the iliopsoas muscle and divides into ascending, transverse, and descending branches at the medial edge of the rectus femoris. The transverse branch enters the fascial cleft between the iliopsoas and rectus femoris muscle and courses along the underside of the rectus, giving off a major branch that reaches the anterolateral proximal femur, near the capsular insertion along the anterior intertrochanteric notch.

The medial circumflex artery crosses the medial portion of the iliopsoas muscle to enter the groove between the iliopsoas and the adductor-pectineus muscle group, wrapping itself completely around the iliopsoas onto its posterior surface, until it reaches the medial side of the proximal femur along its posterior surface. The course of the vessel around the iliopsoas varies with age, but it may be only several millimeters away from the lesser trochanter, particularly in the newborn, and great care must be given to isolate and protect the vessel during any medial-based operative procedures such as the Ludloff or Ferguson approaches. The medial circumflex artery subsequently courses along the intertrochanteric notch posteriorly and eventually comes over the superior portion of

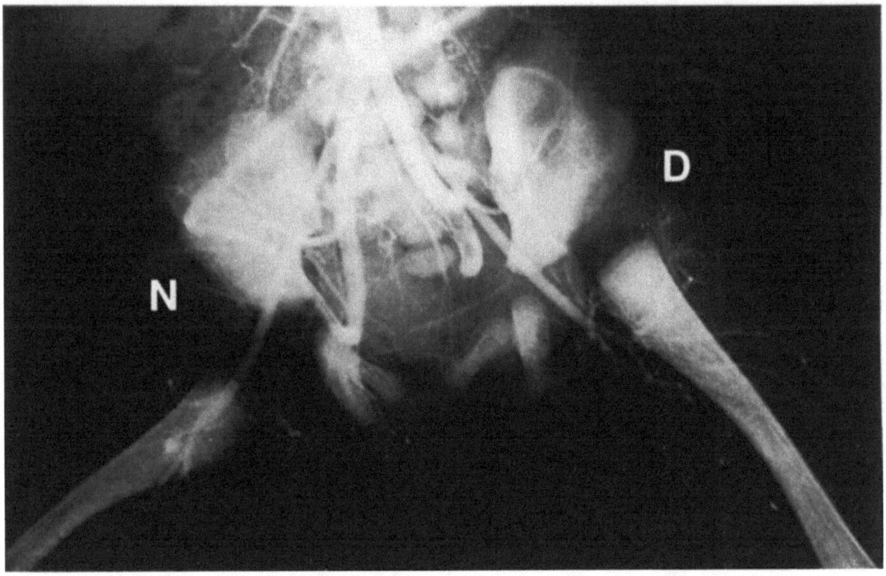

Fig. 29. Postmortem arteriogram showing relatively normal gross distribution of vascularity to dislocated *(D)* hip in a stillborn. Unfortunately the hip could not be removed for more detailed studies (roentgenogram provided by Dr. Neal Small)

the notch to anastomose with terminal portions of the lateral circumflex. As with the lateral circumflex artery, specific patterns of circulation vary with skeletal age and will be discussed in subsequent sections.

Figure 29 illustrates a postmortem arteriogram performed in a child with CDH. As can be seen, despite the dislocation there is adequate filling of the medial and lateral circumflex vessels. However, when compared to the opposite side, there is a definite decrease in the amount of vascularity supplying the region of the dislocated femoral head. While this may be partially a postmortem artifact, this different filling pattern certainly suggests that there may be a mild decrease in the overall circulation to the hip. However, as will be subsequently shown, the microvasculature within the femoral head can be filled with contrast medium even in a severely dislocated hip.

At birth, the growth plate is a transverse, planar structure caudal to both the greater trochanteric and capital femoral regions of the entire femoral chondroepiphysis. Only a small portion of the medial edge of the growth plate is intraarticular at this stage. Blood vessels enter the epiphyseal hyaline cartilage along the intertrochanteric insertion of the capsule both anteriorly and posteriorly. These vessels penetrate the cartilage near its junction with the capsule and do not initially have a significant intraarticular course, inasmuch as the femoral neck has not yet developed. The lateral circumflex artery gives off branches that penetrate the lateral and anterolateral portions of the greater trochanter and much of the anterior portion of the head of the femur along the intertrochanteric notch (Fig. 28). Until the age of 5–6 months, when the femoral neck begins to develop, the lateral circumflex branches supply considerable portions of the anterior capital femoral region of the chondroepiphysis and growth plate. The medial circumflex artery supplies a small anteromedial portion of the growth plate along the capsular insertion and then supplies all the posteromedial and posterolateral growth plate and the posterior chondroepiphysis by penetrating branches along the superior and inferior margins of what will eventually become the femoral neck. In particular, in the superior region of the intertrochanteric groove, several large vessels enter the chondroepiphysis to supply the superior portion of the capital femur. These vessels course to a central area of the femoral head where the ossification center will eventually develop.

Once each arterial branch has entered the chondroepiphysis, it supplies a discrete area of hyaline cartilage or growth cartilage and does not anastomose with other branch terminations within the femoral head or greater trochanter. Infrequently a few vessels supplying the region directly above the growth plate may communicate across the physis with the metaphyseal circulation. These communications are usually arteriosinusoidal, rather than arterial, and tend to occur in the peripheral regions, rather than centrally.

Thus, at birth, even in the dislocatable hip, there is a bipartite circulation to the entire proximal femoral chondroepiphysis, with a minimal contribution by the acetabular artery. The circumflex vessels supply approximately equal portions of both the trochanter and the capital femur and their respective growth plates, with the medial circumflex artery supplying the posterior half and the lateral circumflex artery supplying the anterior half. The medial circumflex artery has a more tortuous course in reaching the hip and is more susceptible to extraarticular compression.

With growth the most significant factor relative to the contributions of the medial and lateral circumflex arteries to the proximal femur is the development of the femoral neck. The formation and elongation of the femoral neck occurs through differential rates of growth within the physis (Ogden, 1974b). These vascular and chondroosseous changes commence at 5–7 months after birth, but appear to be delayed in subluxating and dislocated hips. In the latter circumstance, the development of the secondary ossification center of the femoral head is delayed, and the neck may develop a more anteverted, valgus position. However, this does not appear to change the basic vascular developmental patterns, if the hip has not been treated.

With growth the lateral circumflex branches which had previously penetrated the anterior chondroepiphysis now primarily enter the intracapsular portion of the anterior metaphysis, although a few small anterior branches of the lateral circumflex artery still supply the cartilaginous femoral head, entering peripherally and not crossing the substance of the growth plate. The lateral circumflex artery does increase its contributions to the lateral and anterior portions of the greater trochanter. Similar vascular changes occur posteriorly with many small branches now entering the metaphysis rather than the chondroepiphysis. Several larger branches of the medial circumflex artery become prominent along the superior and inferior margins of the posterior neck and begin to form an intraarticular course, including a microvascular, intraarticular anastomotic arcade, although they are covered by retinacular reflections. The posterosuperior vessels tend to run in small grooves in the cartilaginous contribution to the femoral neck, and sometimes may be completely enclosed in cartilage. The postero-inferior vessels tend to be in loose retinacular reflections that allow them much more mobility in their course along the neck. The posteroinferior branches enter the femoral head on the epiphyseal side of the peripheral segment of the growth plate and distribute to the inferomedial portion of the chondroepiphysis and the medial segment of the proximal part of the capital femoral growth plate. Other branches course along the posterosuperior femoral neck and enter the chondroepiphysis through a fibrofatty area near the femoral head. Neither of these major vascular networks crosses the growth plate substance to reach the chondroepiphysis, but rather courses around the periphery of the growth plate.

The arterial branches most closely associated with development of the secondary ossification center usually stem from the posterosuperior vessels, rather than the posteroinferior or anterior vessels. This dependence on the posterosuperior vessels, which are also quite susceptible to compression during treatment of CDH, may be a major factor in the development of avascular necrosis during treatment. The ossification center is initially associated with one or two of the end-arterial systems of the posterosuperior vessels. By the time it is approximately three to four millimeters in diameter, several end-arterial systems are entering it, allowing anastomosis between posterosuperior and postero-inferior systems. However, the major contributions throughout most of this development, particularly during the critical first 2–3 years of life, come from the posterosuperior branches.

Figure 30 shows a specimen from a fifteen-month-old female with untreated CDH. The vascular injection was done with India ink, using the abdominal aorta. Despite the chronic dislocation, the India ink penetrated into the vessels within the cartilage. The figure demonstrates both the posteroinferior and posterosuperior systems. As can be seen several large vessels are penetrating from the posterosuperior region. In subsequent sections, these vessels supplied the developing ossification center. It should also be noted that there is a large vessel in the intertrochanteric region that traverses between the epiphysis and metaphysis. This is a much larger vessel and was arteriosinusoidal in nature. Despite the chronicity of this dislocation (15 postnatal months), the arterial supply (patency and distribution) was normal.

The most important factor that seems to predispose the proximal end of the femur to vascular insult during treatment for the various types of congenital hip diseases appears to be the transition from a blood supply of multiple small vessels to one more limited in its derivation. At birth, vessels penetrate the chondroepiphysis every few millimeters along the intertrochanteric notch, and each penetrating vessel courses within the chondroepiphysis as an end-arterial system. As the femoral neck develops and elongates, certain vessels assume a more dominant role. Most of the initial anterior epiphyseal and physeal contributions from the lateral circumflex artery regress and the majority of these vessels are redirected to supply anteromedial metaphysis. In contrast, certain branches of the medial circumflex artery along the posterior femoral neck enlarge and elongate commensurate with the elongation of the femoral neck.

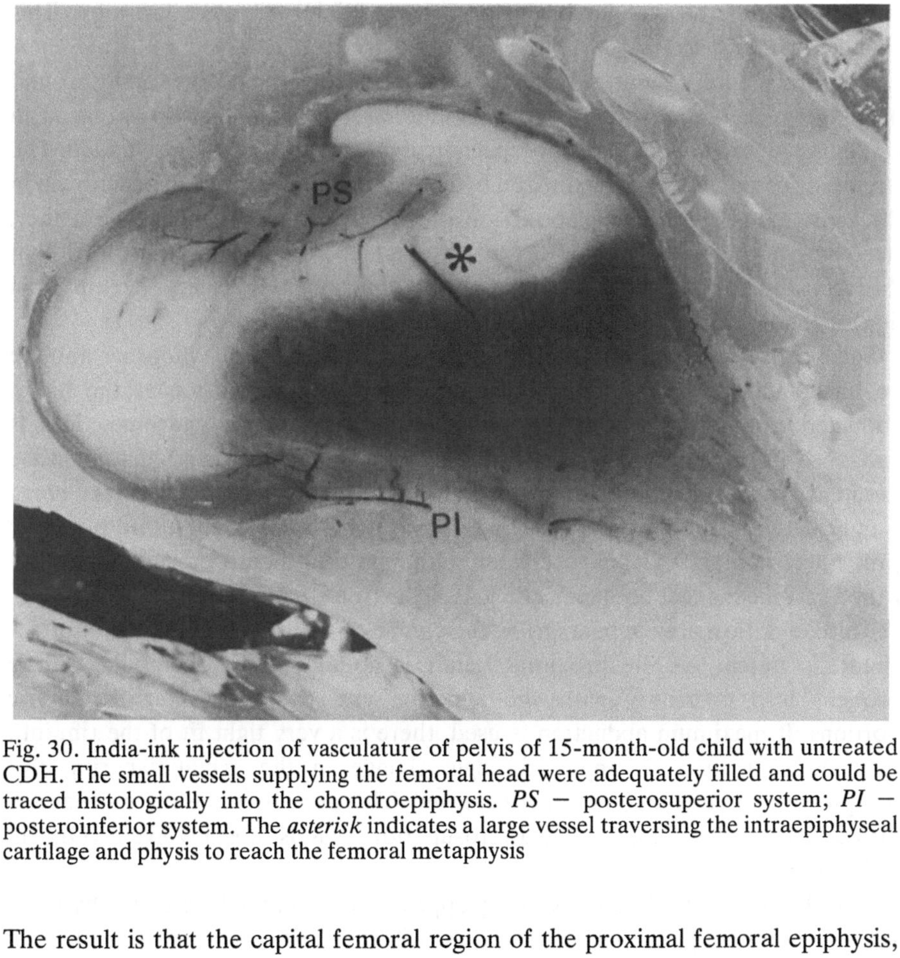

Fig. 30. India-ink injection of vasculature of pelvis of 15-month-old child with untreated CDH. The small vessels supplying the femoral head were adequately filled and could be traced histologically into the chondroepiphysis. *PS* – posterosuperior system; *PI* – posteroinferior system. The *asterisk* indicates a large vessel traversing the intraepiphyseal cartilage and physis to reach the femoral metaphysis

The result is that the capital femoral region of the proximal femoral epiphysis, unlike other epiphyses, is uniquely dependent on a few vessels only for its blood supply. At the microvasculature level, two other important changes are taking place. One is the coalescence of several end-arterial systems of peripheral origins to form the dominant posterosuperior and posteroinferior vessels. Another is the development of intraepiphyseal anastomoses through an intermediary, the secondary ossification center.

During the transition phase from multiple to limited vessels the capital femoral epiphysis is extremely susceptible to vascular compromise, particularly if there is any alteration in the anatomy. Occlusion of a small vessel along the intertrochanteric groove in the first few months of life might affect only a small area, whereas occlusion of a single vessel such as the posterosuperior branch in a slightly older child could have a profound effect on subsequent development of the proximal femur. Furthermore, since the blood supply begins as a multiple small vessel system, vascular compromise severe enough to cause the growth changes seen in avascular necrosis in congenital hip disease implies occlusion of vessels of significant size, rather than multiple small vessels. In the child treated during the first few weeks of life who eventually develops avascular necrosis, the implication must be that the occlusion occurred external to the hip joint. This may occur in several areas.

First, the medial circumflex artery, as it courses toward and eventually around the iliopsoas tendon, is subjected to undue stretch when the hip is placed in maximum abduction and flexion, especially if internal rotation is also added. The stretching of the vessel is maximized by abduction, although it can occur even in the hip treated by minimal abduction but marked internal rotation. Further, stretching of the medial circumflex artery may occur because of translocation of the iliopsoas tendon from its normal anatomic position when the hip is in neutral, to other positions when the hip is flexed and abducted.

Second, as the medial circumflex artery courses between the iliopsoas and the pectineus-adductor group, it may be subjected to compression as the hip is abducted, similar to a scalenus anticus (thoracic outlet) syndrome. This is enhanced in the child that has a contracture in the pectineus-adductor muscle group. Marked abduction may also result in the medial circumflex artery being caught between the iliopsoas tendon and the pubic ramus. These are potential sites for temporary vascular occlusion, although treatment in a rigid immobilization cast means that occlusion can feasibly exist for many weeks.

Third, a critical area appears to be the course of the vessels along the intertrochanteric notch. As the proximal femur is abducted, the acetabular rim is brought into proximity with the superior and posterior intertrochanteric portions. If maximum abduction is used, there is a very tight fit of the rim into the notch. If there is any pathologic change in the acetabular rim, this compressive force is undoubtedly increased. This appears to be the mechanism of occlusion when only the posterosuperior vessels are involved (Ogden, 1974b).

Fourth, the lateral circumflex artery appears to be minimally affected by these various treatment positions. However, the effective anastomosis with the medial circumflex artery across the superior portion of the intertrochanteric notch appears to be minimal and not capable of assuming a dominant role in the case of vascular compromise.

Another important point is the relationship of the blood vessels to the joint capsule. Along the intertrochanteric notch the blood vessels, both veins and arteries, are external to the joint capsule. Vessels traverse the capsule at the level of the insertion into the cartilage of the intertrochanteric notch. A few small branches course within the capsule itself, but these small vessels have no role in the blood supply of the proximal femur. Therefore, anterior or posterior capsulotomy, if done carefully, should not affect the blood supply of the proximal part of the femur, as long as the underlying and anatomically separate anterior, posterosuperior and posteroinferior vessels are not damaged, and as long as the capsular incision is not carried down to the intertrochanteric notch. An anterior approach to the hip is less likely to damage the major sources of blood supply. The medial circumflex artery, as it courses around the iliopsoas tendon, is also susceptible to damage during surgery, particularly if one uses a medial approach and transects the tendon near its insertion into the lesser trochanter. Due to the usual anteverted, mild valgus position of the proximal femur, one should remember that the posteroinferior vessels may be in the fibrofatty tissue just underneath the iliopsoas tendon and just above the lesser trochanter. Again, great care should be taken to try to avoid damaging these vessels when doing a capsulotomy from this approach.

Summary and Conclusions

Types of Dislocation

Classification may be based upon two criteria – primary causes and secondary changes. From an etiologic standpoint congenital hip disease may be classified as teratologic or typical. The use of these terms implies known etiology, usually of a neurologic nature, versus an idiopathic problem that probably arises due to intrauterine positioning and physiologic changes accompanying the last trimester of pregnancy (capsular response to hormonal changes). The teratologic hip frequently is severely subluxated or completely dislocated at birth, and may worsen during the postnatal period due to continued abnormal forces particularly if the deformity is sequential to a neurologic disorder. A child with a high-level myelomeningocoele may have significant deformity at birth, whereas a child with a lower-level myelomeningocoele may not begin to manifest hip deformity until the postnatal period. Similarly the teratologic hip of a child with cerebral palsy will occur in a hip that has developed normally throughout gestation, and only begins to deform postnatally in accord with the type of palsy (e.g., flaccid versus spastic) and degree of muscular involvement. In contrast the typical hip "dislocation" is only rarely truly dislocated. In reality this type of hip is unstable in some positions and stable in others. However, it should be "reducible" in appropriate positions of flexion and abduction. It should be realized that the arbitrary terms "typical" and "teratologic" refer only to etiology, and should not be equated with the degree of deformity.

From an anatomic standpoint congenital hip disease may be grouped into three types:

Type 1: This hip probably comprises 80%–90% of the CDH classification and may be defined as a subluxatable or positionally unstable hip. There usually are mild marginal changes in the acetabulum, while the femoral head is anteverted but spherically normal. There are mild adduction and flexion contractures attributable to the muscles (adductors), although much of the soft tissue tightness may be in the anterior and inferior joint capsule. If left untreated this is probably the type of hip that may progress to more severe deformity, or, more likely, may become the subluxated/anteverted hip of the older child. This type of hip probably would not manifest an Ortolani sign, but would exhibit lack of abduction.

Type 2: This hip, which can be considered subluxated, will begin to show loss of sphericity of the femoral head as well as anteversion. Due to pressure from different portions of the femoral head the acetabulum is more shallow, has a significant narrowing of the anterior margin and is beginning to show superior and posterior marginal deformities, primarily eversion of the labrum. The eversion soft tissue changes are accompanied by osseous changes – the acetabular roof fails to ossify laterally, leading to increased acetabular acclivity, which is an early roentgenographic sign. If untreated this hip probably progresses to a more severe subluxation or even complete dislocation. The hip usually has more severe flexion and adduction contractures, and as the extensor/abductor groups (especially gluteus medius and minimus) become more active postnatally, they may pull the positionally susceptible proximal femur superiorly and/or posteriorly, accentuating the marginal eversion. During this stage the first traces of inversion of the limbus may be discerned. It appears that inversion may not be an abrupt phenomenon, but rather a gradual process of hypertrophy and ingrowth of that portion of the fibrocartilaginous labrum adjacent to the hyaline cartilage. At this stage the inversional hypertrophy, which is associated with eversion of most of the labrum, is undoubtedly reversible. This type of hip probably exhibits a "clicking" sensation during an Ortolani maneuver, as well as loss of full abduction.

Type 3: This hip is the most severely involved, with significant deformation of the acetabular margin and femoral head, and a posterosuperior displacement of the head to form a false acetabulum by eversion of the labrum. Inversional hypertrophy of the fibrocartilage to form the limbus posterosuperiorly causes the acetabulum to be more incongruent relative to the femoral head. Further, the more hypertrophied the limbus, the more pressure it will apply to the femoral head to cause secondary indentations and continued loss of sphericity. The ligamentum capitis femoris is elongated, but it is also pulled up from its normal origin, bringing along the transverse acetabular ligament, which also compromises acetabular volume and further precludes reduction. During the first 24–48 hours there is frequently sufficient laxity to manifest a "clunking" sensation with on Ortolani maneuver, with a concomitant dislocation during the Barlow maneuver.

While the less severe anatomic types appear to be associated with typical CDH, and the more severe anatomic changes with teratologic CDH, the findings in this study strongly suggest that there is an overlap of pathologic change in this concatenate disease. Further, many teratologic dislocations occur postnatally in previously normal hips, a situation not unlike the untreated typical CDH found only after the child begins ambulation. The major differences between typical and teratologic CDH are the chronicity and degree of muscular deforming forces, and the time of dislocation (which will be discussed subsequently). Because each etiologic type has at least three recognizable anatomic types, it is imperative that the treating physician define as accurately as possible the pathologic changes and direct treatment appropriately.

Time of Dislocation

The exact onset of any subluxation or dislocation is difficult to ascertain. Undoubtedly it is a gradual process. During the intrauterine period anatomic changes may occur very rapidly because of the growth acceleration of the fetus. In contrast, anatomicopathologic changes occur more slowly during the postnatal period because of relatively decreased rates of growth. This study has suggested that a stage of subluxation (types 1 and 2), often prolonged, exists before a true dislocation (type 3) is finally established. Subluxation probably can begin anytime after the tenth to twelfth intrauterine week, after the acetabular, femoral and capsular components of the hip joint have become differentiated. The hip that is severely deformed at birth probably falls into the teratologic group, with abnormalities such as myelomeningocoele, arthrogryposis and urinary tract abnormalities associated with oligohydraminos being major primary factors. However, the child presenting as a frank breech, with hyperextended knees, also may exhibit significant deformity, and yet have no primary factors other than intrauterine position. In both situations the rapid growth of the fetus causes type 2 or 3 structural deformities by the time of birth. Similarly, intrauterine positioning and maternal/fetal physiologic changes appear to act in utero to create the conditions leading to the most common types of CDH (types 1 and 2), which are characterized by positional instability and contractures. Therefore, in all types of CDH, most, if not all, predisposing factors have caused some anatomic change during the prenatal period.

Since many of the secondary changes – capsular distension, acetabular marginal deformity, femoral anteversion and soft tissue contractures – associated with types 1 and 2 persist during the postnatal period, and because other muscular forces (e.g., glutei) become more prominent, the gradual development of the type 3 dislocation may occur. The high occurrence of type 3 CDH in certain ethnic groups with characteristic ways of wrapping the neonates undoubtedly gradually converts a susceptible, or even normal hip into a severe dislocation by forcing the hip into positions not conducive to normal postnatal development. The newborn hip structurally and functionally does not seem capable of being placed in extension. Efforts to do this in stillborn hips only cause the femoral head to subluxate posterosuperiorly. Often has it been suggested that weight-bearing may play a role, but as Somerville has shown, it is more likely that the only effect of weight-bearing is to facilitate the diagnosis since the awkward gait becomes obvious to the parents. The major primary factors acting postnatally to cause or increase anatomicopathologic changes appear to be the functional development of the hip extensor/abductor muscle group and the assumption of hip extension.

Changes in the Proximal Femur

Anteversion seems to be the primary problem affecting the proximal femur that plays a dominant role in subluxation and dislocation. Le Damany (1908) suggested that the entire sequence of events eventuating in dislocation resulted from anteversion. In more recent years Badgley (1943–1949) produced additional evidence that anteversion was an important factor. As shown in this study the in utero position of the femoral head places eccentric rather than central pressures on the acetabular margins. Anteversion seems to enhance the probability of this femoral head/acetabular eccentricity. Unfortunately treatment based only on correction of anteversion by femoral osteotomy has never proved to be entirely satisfactory. On the basis of the observations in this study there is a very obvious answer. Redirecting the femoral head into a more acceptable anatomic position does not correct the secondary changes which have already occurred in the acetabulum, particularly in the older child, and it may be necessary to consider some type of pelvic osteotomy in conjunction with femoral surgery (although not necessarily as a one-stage surgical procedure). These interrelated changes exist in both subluxated (type 2) and dislocated (type 3) hips.

It is extremely important to realize that this concatenation of anatomico-pathologic changes affects both sides of the hip joint, and may necessitate surgical endeavors directed at both sides, rather than an emphasis on either pelvic osteotomy or femoral derotation osteotomy.

In many dislocated hips there were major changes in the overall contours of the femoral heads, particularly in the older children. These changes were associated with considerable incongruity between proximal femur and acetabulum, and they certainly decreased the likelihood of concentric reduction. The longer the hip was dislocated, the greater were the deformities of the proximal femur. Further, the increased anteversion was usually associated with increased neck/shaft angulation, leading to severe valgus deformity. The most severely involved hip in this study had valgus beyond 180° and anteversion beyond 90°.

Changes in the Acetabulum

The major changes which occur in the acetabulum, both prenatally and postnatally, are marginal deformations that create a shallow, seemingly anteverted acetabulum. The most characteristic change was narrowing or even complete absence of the anterior wall of the acetabulum. This involved both the fibrocartilaginous labrum as well as the articular hyaline cartilage. The deformity could be correlated easily with deforming pressure from the eccentrically placed femoral head. The superior and posterior walls showed narrowing of the fibrocartilaginous labrum, although some cases showed widening posteriorly. The labrum and articular surface usually showed some degree of eversion, again in direct association with the eccentric position of the femoral head. These acetabular changes thus appeared to be secondary (adaptational) responses to the anteversion and intrauterine position of the hip, rather than primary acetabular dysplasia.

The superior labral eversion changes noted on gross examination correlated with similar acclivity changes on roentgenography. In early stages of fetal hip development the ossified portion of the roof is more transverse than oblique. However, as the acetabulum grows and as eccentrically lateralized pressure from the anteverted, subluxating femoral head is applied, there are gradual changes that may lead to a roentgenographically evident increased obliquity of the entire osseous roof, or of a localized lateral section. But, as noted in several of the specimens, the osseous changes may be minimal when compared to significant cartilaginous deformation. Again, these osseous changes are simply a secondary response to adjacent cartilage changes and eccentrically applied pressure from the femoral head.

The limbus presents a major impediment to reduction, especially in the older child. Unfortunately its mechanism of formation has been poorly understood. It has often been attributed to modalities of conservative treatment used preceding any open reduction. However, several examples were encountered in newborns, which makes it seem unlikely that treatment methods play a primary role, although a secondary adaptational role cannot be totally discounted in the older patient. From the current studies it appears that the limbus is, like the other alterations in the acetabulum, a secondary response to eccentric pressure. Several hips showed both eversion and beginning inversion of the labrum. The inversion was occurring at the margin of the fibro- and hyaline cartilage, along its posterosuperior portion. This strongly suggests that inversion may be a gradual, not an abrupt, change, and that this tissue is biologically quite plastic. This can be readily observed when doing arthrography under fluoroscopy – some degree of inversion of the limbus of the dislocated hip flattens out when the hip is reduced. This structure becomes more rigid the longer the hip remains dislocated, and it is more likely that it may have to be removed surgically to accomplish reduction. *Arthrography* must be considered an essential part of CDH treatment, since the surgeon must be aware of the extent of deformity of the acetabular margins. We prefer to do this only after preliminary traction of at least two weeks duration.

An often neglected structure in discussing CDH is the transverse acetabular ligament which crosses the inferior acetabulum. This ligament is in direct continuity with the anterior and posterior fibrocartilaginous labrum, and probably should be considered as an integral part of the labrum, rather than a discrete ligament. As the proximal femur is displaced superiorly, this structure is also pulled superiorly and contracts, effectively blocking the lower portion of the acetabulum and contributing to incongruent reduction. Again, it may be necessary to excise this tissue to accomplish an effective reduction.

In the examples of subluxation in the older child, the characteristic findings were lack of an anterior acetabular wall in conjunction with an anteverted femoral head showing some mild posteromedial flattening. The superior and posterior walls were somewhat everted and widened which contributed to the appearance of anteversion of the acetabulum. Pelvic osteotomy, as described by Salter, very effectively improved the acetabular position, but tended to externally rotate the femora, suggesting that derotation osteotomy may also be necessary in many cases.

Direction of Dislocation

There is continuing controversy about the exact direction in which dislocation occurs. If one conceives of CDH as a progressive, rather than abrupt, deformity, a better understanding of the direction of displacement is much easier. Based on the conclusions of Somerville and the observations in this study, it appears that the initial anterior wall deficiency and superior marginal deficiency, plus the intrauterine hip flexion (and neonatal flexion contracture) cause the proximal femur to initially be displaced anterosuperiorly. However, as previously described, the posterior wall is also beginning to deform. When the hip gradually assumes the extended position, muscular forces and capsular contractures enhance a migration from anterosuperior to posterosuperior. In the severely intrauterine dislocation (type 3) this posterior displacement may occur even when the hip is flexed. In most cases there is superior displacement. The variation occurs in the amount of associated anterior or posterior displacement, with posterior displacement being most characteristic in the postnatal phase, and anterior displacement in the prenatal phase.

Blood Supply

From the few cases that I could study in sufficient detail, the gross patterns of distribution of the blood supply to the proximal femur, both extraarticular and intraepiphyseal, are the same as the normal hip. However, relationships to various structures change as the hip displaces. In particular the shift of the iliopsoas increases risk of compression of the main trunk of the medial circumflex artery as it wraps itself around the tendon, and the development of the labrum to a more hypertrophic structure superiorly and posteriorly enhances risk of occlusion of the vessels along the posterior intertrochanteric notch. Avascular necrosis is a serious and undoubtedly avoidable complication. Awareness of patterns of circulation and how they might be compromised by nonoperative or operative measures is essential.

Ossification Center

While a minimal degree of asymmetry of development of the secondary ossification centers may be within the limits of biologic variation, any retardation of the development of the ossific nucleus should make one suspicious of CDH. While the ossification centers usually appear at reasonably predictable times (approximately 4–6 month postpartum) the eccentric pressures of the subluxating or dislocated hip may not impart sufficient joint reaction forces to stimulate development of the nucleus at its normal time. However, once the hip is being treated appropriately, the ossification center usually rapidly appears and/or enlarges until symmetry is attained. Any significant delay in appearance, fragmentation or irregularity should suggest vascular compromise and the need to follow the patient through skeletal maturation, since epiphyseal and physeal growth abnormalities may not occur until the adolescent growth spurt.

Acknowledgement

I would like to gratefully acknowledge the cooperation of the Departments of Anatomy of Yale University, the University of Vermont, and St. Louis University, Joan Walker of MacMaster University, Dr. Aloysio Campos da Paz of Brasilia and Dr. Ignacio Ponseti of the University of Iowa, for their contributions of case materials that added immeasurably to this study.

References

Campos da Paz, A.: Ital. J. Orth. Traum. **2,** 261 (1976)
Chung, S. M.: J. Bone Joint Surg. **58-A,** 961 (1976)
Crelin, E. S.: Yale J. Biol. Med. **49,** 109 (1976)
Dunn, P. M.: Clin. Orthop. **119,** 11 (1976a)
Dunn, P. M.: Clin. Orthop. **119,** 23 (1976b)
Fairbank, H.: Brit. J. Surg. **17,** 380 (1930)
Hennemann, D.: Endocrinology **83,** 678 (1968)
Laurenson, R. D.: J. Bone Joint Surg. **46-A,** 283 (1964)
Laurenson, R. D.: J. Bone Joint Surg. **47-A,** 975 (1965)
LeVeuf, J.: J. Bone Joint Surg. **29,** 149 (1947)
McKibbin, B.: J. Bone Joint Surg. **52-B,** 148 (1970
Michelsson, J. E., Langenskiold, A.: J. Bone Joint Surg. **54-A,** 1177 (1972)
Milgram, J. W., Tachdjian, M. O.: Clin. Orthop. **119,** 107 (1976)
Nishimura, H.: In Congenital Malformations. Amsterdam: Excerpta Medica 1970
Ogden, J. A.: J. Bone Joint Surg. **56-A,** 941 (1974a)
Ogden, J. A.: In The Hip. St. Louis: C. V. Mosby Co. 1974b
Ogden, J. A., Jensen, P.: Radiology **119,** 189 (1976)
Ralis, Z., McKibbin, B.: J. Bone Joint Surg. **55-B,** 780 (1973)
Smith, W. S., Lieberg, O., Gobelsman, U.: Clin. Orthop. **88,** 56 (1972)
Somerville, E. W.: J. Bone Joint Surg. **35-B,** 568 (1953)
Stanisavljevic, S., Mitchell, C. L.: J. Bone Joint Surg. **45-A,** 1147 (1963)
Stanisavljevic, S.: Congenital Hip Pathology in the Newborn. Baltimore: Williams and Wilkins Co. 1964

Development and Clinical Importance of the Dysplastic Acetabulum

W. Dega*

A. The Fetal Acetabulum

I. The Structural Components of the Normal Fetal Acetabulum

During the first three embryonic months, i.e., during the period of organogenesis, all the structural components of the acetabulum are formed, and the way is thus prepared for further fetal development. The clinical importance of fetal development of the hip lies in the fact that these structural components are formed while the femur is flexed, whereas Homo erectus will use his hip joint in extension. The child is unable to do this during the first year of life. His first attempts at crawling are made at 3–4 months of age, using all four extremities. The first walking attempts, beginning at the end of the first year, are carried out with a distinct flexion of the hip and knee joints.

The conflict between the anatomic structure of the hip joint and its later functional demands becomes manifest during the perinatal period, parturition representing the midpoint.

P. Le Damany of Rennes (1905) was probably the first to draw attention to this conflict. His investigations were pursued by Graf (1909) and later by R. J. Harrenstein of Amsterdam (1928) who referred to a "period of danger" in the formation of the hip joint.

These extremely interesting studies led me to examine the data of le Damany, Graf and Harrenstein with regard to our own case material. To this end, since 1926 I have performed anatomic and anthropometric examinations of 100 human stillborn fetuses aged 4–9 months. My first results were published in 1929.

In general, my findings agree with those of the above-mentioned authors. Additionally, however, my studies have yielded some interesting contributions to the pathogenesis of hip dysplasia and its clinical consequences for prevention and early treatment (1930, 1932). The results of my studies may be briefly summarized as follows: In 200 acetabula examined, the aperture was more com-

* Institute for Orthopaedics and Rehabilitation, Poznàn, Poland

monly round in younger fetuses, more often ovoid in older fetuses (on the average 29% round, 57% vertically ovoid, and in 16% horizontally ovoid).

The limbus of the acetabulum (Fig. 1) has a wide base and a thin sharp border. It is therefore triangular in cross section. The base abuts on and is continuous with the cartilaginous border of the acetabulum. Its height decreases with the age of the fetus, relatively more so in its posterior segment than anteriorly.

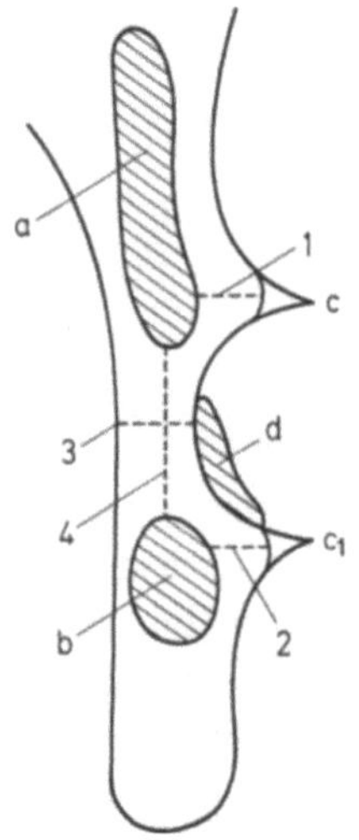

Fig. 1. Cross section of the acetabulum through the anterior-superior spine of the ilium and the ischial tuberosity. *a* Ossification center of ilium. *b* Ossification center of ischium c, c_1 Acetabular lip. *d* Fat pad. *1, 2* Cartilaginous rim of acetabulum. *3* Thickness of cartilaginous floor of acetabulum. *4* Triradiate carilage

The depth of the acetabulum diminishes in the course of fetal growth. At 4–5 months the acetabulum completely surrounds the head of the femur. Flattening out begins in the 6th or 7th month. The floor of the acetabulum does not take part in this process, its thickness remaining proportionally constant during the entire fetal period. The inclination of the acetabulum, inferiorly and anteriorly, becomes steeper with growth of the fetus. The inferior angle of inclination averages 29° in the 6th or 7th fetal month, 26° in the 7th or 8th month, 25° in the 8th or 9th month, and increases at birth to 27°.

The anterior angle of inclination begins later to decrease somewhat: in the 7th month it is 30°, in the 8th month 28°, in the 9th month 26°, and at birth it averages 27°.

Sexual distinctions are noticeable in the angle of the oblique plane of the acetabular aperture, especially in the inferior acetabular angle, which is several degrees steeper in the female fetus than in the male.

The progressive decrease in the depth of the acetabulum and the vertical position of the plane of the acetabular aperture proceed synchronously with anteversion of the neck of the femur.

According to our measurements anteversion increases from about 0° in the 4th or 5th fetal month to an average of about 28° in male newborns and about 34° in females.

The angles of the acetabulum and of the neck of the femur are of no consequence in the prenatal period. They become important only in newborns and infants.

II. The Mode of Origin of Dysplasia of the Acetabulum

Let us now consider the articular axes of the hip in the prenatal position of flexion of the thigh. A cross section (Fig. 2) through the middle of the hip joints and parallel to the plane of the inlet of the minor pelvis of a 9-month-old fetus shows that the axis of the femoral neck and a line drawn perpendicular to the midpoint of the plane of the acetabular aperture, i.e., the acetabular axis, can be superimposed. In the fetal position, therefore, the head of the femur is well seated in the acetabulum. At parturition the newborn is released from the flexed position. Deflexion of the legs begins, i.e., fetal flexion changes to postnatal extension.

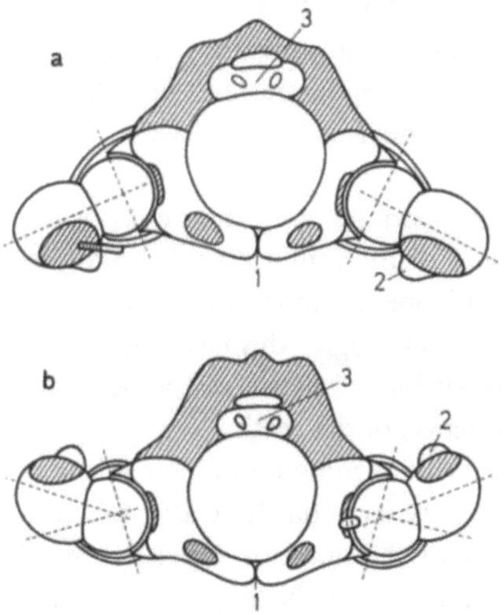

Fig. 2. Cross section of the hip joints parallel to the plane of the pelvic inlet of a 9-month fetus. (a) Normal intrauterine flexion of the hips. (b) Theoretical full extension of the hip. *1* Symphysis pubis. *2* Lesser trochanter. *3* Sacrum

The joint capsule with its ligaments, which has likewise developed in the fetal flexed position of the hip, counteracts abrupt extension of the hip, ensuring that deflexion takes place slowly. This is of fundamental importance for postnatal prevention of hip dislocation.

If one removes the joint capsule together with its ligaments and surrounding muscles and positions the head of the fully extended femur in the acetabulum,

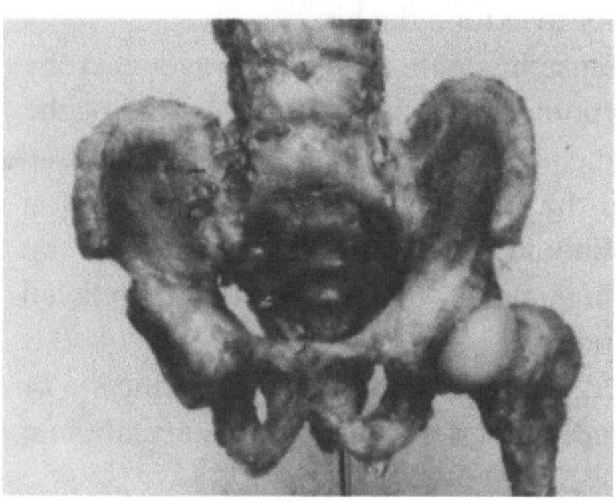

Fig. 3. Anatomic specimen of the pelvis of a normal neonate. Joint capsule is removed. Femur in extension. Anterior prominence of the femoral head

the axes of the acetabulum and neck of the femur intersect. The head of the femur protrudes anteriorly from the acetabulum (Fig. 3). The greater the anteversion of the femoral neck, the more the head of the femur will be exposed anteriorly; therefore its contact surface with the acetabulum is decreased with resulting instability.

Associated with this state are the shallowness and steepness of the acetabulum, which becomes noticeable in the final fetal months. From this one must conclude that there is an insufficient congruence of the hip joint at the time of birth. Harrenstein calls this the period of physiologic danger of the hip joint.

Paradoxically, nowadays one could speak of a physiologic or, even better, of an anthropologic dysplasia of the hip joint in the newborn. The borderline between the physiologic and the pathologic state is so labile that if the pathologic boundary is not crossed, there is regression back to the norm in the first few months after birth, i.e., the acetabulum again becomes deeper and less slanted and the increased anteversion of the neck of the femur decreases, finally reaching in adults a value of about 12°.

However, should one of these three labile components, i.e., the depth or the inclination of the acetabulum or the anteversion of the femoral neck, retain its increased value at the time of birth or should one or more of these values increase even further, then the so-called physiologic dysplasia becomes pathologic. The well-known clinical symptoms of hip dysplasia of the newborn appear, such as Ortolani's sign and limited abduction of the thigh.

Since the three components interact, all *three* will become pathologic if one of them does. Thus increased anteversion contributes secondarily to the acetabulum's becoming shallow and to the hypotrophy of the anterior superior rim of the acetabulum, which in turns increases the acclivity of the upper part of the acetabulum.

III. The Influence of Mechanical Factors on the Shape of the Fetal Acetabulum

In the fetal position, the iliofemoral ligament originates at the lower part of the anterior inferior spine of the ilium and strengthens the anterior part of the joint capsule. It acts in opposition to any attempt to extend the hip.

If the force of extension is great, the tense ligament exerts leverage whereby its distal point of attachment acts as a hypomochlion. It presses the head of the femur against the anteriosuperior rim of the acetabulum.

In the fetal flexed position of the hip the joint capsule and the iliofemoral ligament are in maximum relaxation. Should a force (e.g., pressure of the uterine wall) be brought to bear on the thigh along the femoral axis, the relaxed iliofemoral ligament will exert no counteraction.

If, however, additional forces connected with either abduction or adduction or internal or external rotation are introduced, other deformities of the acetabulum can arise.

As a result of flexion of the hip the knee joint is facing superiorly while the posterior aspect of the femur with the lesser trochanter is facing anteriorly. External rotation tightens the joint capsule. The neck of the femur impinges on the anterior limbus when the lower limb is placed in adduction and external rotation and the knee is pressed against the body of the fetus. The head of the femur presses against the posterior rim of the acetabulum, deflecting the posterior limbus backward.

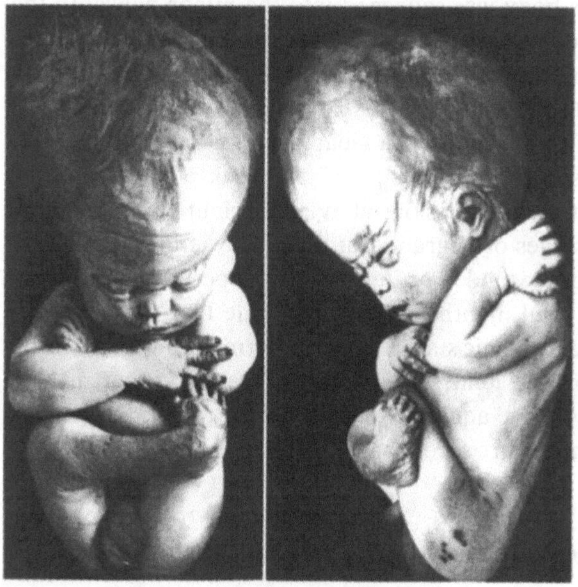

a b

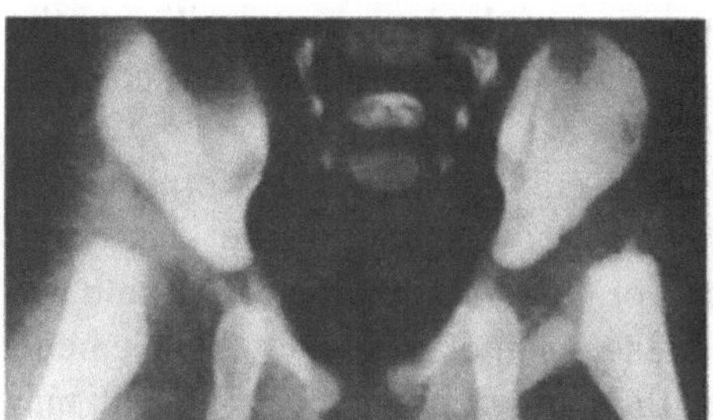

c

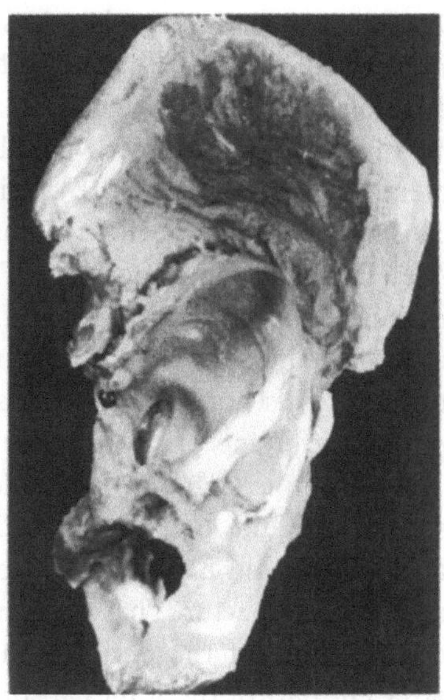

Fig. 4. Specimens from the collection of R. Bernbeck. (Kinderorthopädie. Stuttgart: Georg Thieme, 1954)

d

Do these theoretical considerations correspond to reality? In the embryonic period the embryo is surrounded on all sides by amniotic fluid. It is thus protected against the influence of any local pressure. In the fetal period, under normal conditions, the pressure of the uterus is increasingly distributed over the entire surface of the fetus. However, deviations in the position of the fetus may occur, with pathologic consequences. An example of this has been furnished by R. Bernbeck from his collection.

A mature stillborn fetus with massive internal hydrocephalus (complete obstruction of the cerebral aqueduct) is shown in Figure 4: The head of the fetus (Fig. 4a) was so large that its body was squeezed into the minor pelvis. In the lateral view (Fig. 4b) one observes hyperflexion of the hips, clubfeet, and necrotic areas of skin indicating abnormal effects of pressure. Radiography of the hip showed bilateral dislocations (Fig. 4c).

The anatomic specimen (Fig. 4d) showed a clear depression in the anteriosuperior acetabular rim, caused by the pressure of the neck of the femur. In addition, one can distinguish three impressions above the primitive acetabulum. They correspond with three stages of migration of the dislocated femoral head. The joint capsule is accordingly extended posteriorly and superiorly. This dislocation took place during the fetal months. One can assume that the hip joints were normal in the primitive embryonic stage. Their malformation was the result of external pressure acting on the joints. This fetus had several other malformations. Obstruction of the cerebral aqueduct was, however, the primary deformity. The dislocations of the hips were secondary.

IV. Effect of Ultraphysiologic Positions of the Lower Limb on the Shape of the Acetabulum

There are deviations in the physiologic position of the lower extremities of the fetus which cannot be called pathologic. Chandler calls them "ultraphysiologic" positions.

An example from my own collection is an 8-month-old stillborn fetus with its membranes (Fig. 5a and b). His lower limb was extended at the knee joint, causing hyperflexion with external rotation of the hip joint. The lower limb was in an ultraphysiologic position. This can be the result of normal fetal movements in the uterus, which are present from the 5th month of pregnancy. The limb may meet with an obstacle, e.g., the umbilical cord, and thus be prevented from returning to its normal flexed position. This ultraphysiologic position can exert pathologic effects on the acetabulum if it becomes fixed.

An example from my own collection is the anatomic specimen of a fetal pelvis shown in Figure 6. There is a distinct depression in the anterior limbus of the acetabulum and a posterior displacement of the posterior acetabular rim. The acetabular aperture has become horizontally ovoid. A well-defined bony condensation of the periosteum is seen on the neck of the femur, and in the adjacent part of the joint capsule a fold is noted. The bony condensation at the a

b

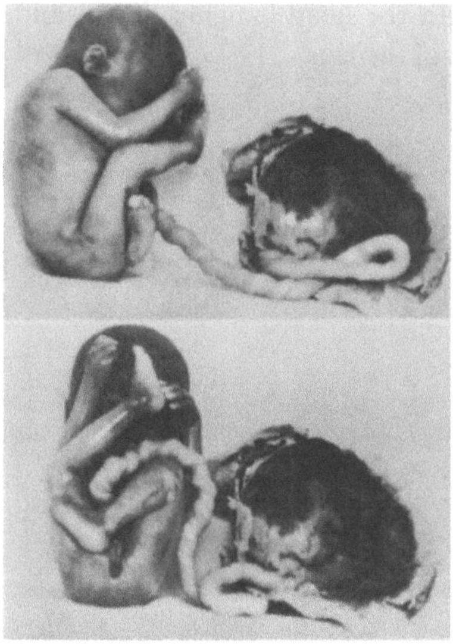

Fig. 5a and b. Eight-month fetus with ultraphysiologic position of right leg. The fetus was stillborn

neck of the femur conforms to the depression of the acetabular rim in flexion and adduction of the femur.

Figure 7, another case from my collection, shows the acetabulum of a fetus with its membranes, whose limb was in the ultraphysiologic position (see Fig. 5). The anterior limbus is completely inverted in the direction of the acetabulum; its posterior rim is clearly displaced posteriorly. The acetabular aperture has lost its round shape and resembles a human ear, a characteristic alteration in dysplasia of the hip.

One can well imagine that these abnormalities of the anterosuperior rim of the acetabulum threaten to reduce the stability of the hip when the extremely abducted femur is in extension or in the Lorenz I position. Hence, the following clinical conclusions as regards prevention: The hips of newborns and infants should be protected from extreme extension as well as from abrupt (e.g.,

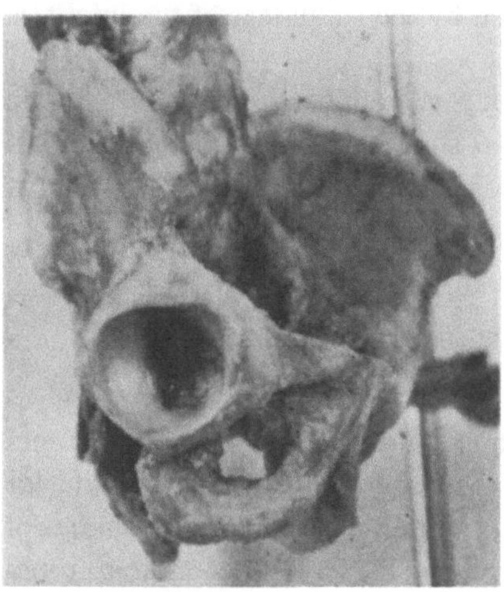

Fig. 6. Slight depression in anterior limbus; the posterior limbus is inverted. (Specimen from author's own collection)

parturition or holding the child by the feet with the head hanging down) and chronic extension (e.g., mummy-like wrappings of the legs).

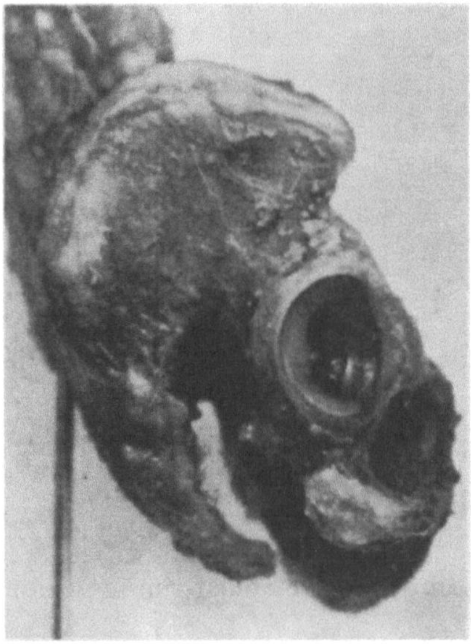

Fig. 7. Total inversion of the anterior limbus; the posterior limbus is turned backward. (Specimen from author's own collection)

B. The Acetabulum After Birth

The fetal position of the hips is responsible for the clinically well-known physiologic contracture of the infant hip after birth.

Although the child tries to fight against this contracture by kicking movements, his extremities are not sufficiently developed to accept the specific functions provided for them. Portmann (cited in F. Becker) speaks of an additional "extra-uterine fetal period" which lasts about 9 months. H. Büschelberger points out that the maternal abdomen clasped by the small legs of the infant, is the proper place for his further development.

As a matter of fact, those countries where it is custom for the mother to tie the child to her body during her daily occupations show the lowest incidence of hip dislocations. As for the rest of us, abduction treatment instituted early must substitute for the flexion-abduction position at the maternal abdomen.

I. Spontaneous Disappearance of Dysplasia

In the majority of infants the head of the femur automatically occupies its functionally correct position in the acetabulum, thereby creating the potential for spontaneous repair of prenatal limbus defects as well as of minor deformities of the acetabulum, even in the presence of clinically evident symptoms of a dysplastic hip, such as Ortoloni's sign. This agrees with our statistical studies of 36,000 newborns which show that hip dysplasias are found in 4% of newborns, while dislocations amounted to about 0.2%. It is easy to imagine that acetabular defects of the type shown in Figure 6 can be self-correcting. The fetal defect shown in Figure 7 is much less likely to correct itself spontaneously.

II. Dysplasia With Partial Progressive Dislocation

If hip dysplasia is left untreated, the deformed acetabulum will become permanent. In time it will result in a joint malformation which in its turn will bring about the appearance of additional secondary deformities. A critical time for the dysplastic hip is the period when the child begins to walk and weight-bearing begins to occur at the hip.

The previously established dysplasia without dislocation will easily progress to a dysplasia with dislocation. The head of the femur presses in a cranial direction, increasing the atrophy of the acetabular lip. The acclivity of the acetabulum increases. The limbus, following the head of the femur, is everted superiorly. The ligament of the head of the femur becomes hypertrophic and pulls the transverse ligament in the direction of the acetabulum. The now empty floor of the acetabulum is filled by an enlarged pad of fibrofatty tissue, the Haversion fat pad. The osseous floor of the acetabulum becomes thickened and appears in the roentgenogram as a condensation of Köhler's "tear drop".

The head of the femur finally settles upon the superior rim of the acetabulum which it compresses either anteriorly or posteriorly with lesser or greater lateral displacement.

III. Dysplasia With Full Dislocation

a) The Slowly Progressing Form

In the slowly progressing form of dysplasia the position of the femoral head at the edge of the acetabulum may – even after many years – prove to be transitional. The femoral head then begins to migrate and leaves the acetabulum. A subluxation becomes a dislocation.

The acetabulum is expanded lengthwise and exhibits slight hourglass-shaped depressions, marking the stage-by-stage migration of the femoral head.

The changes in the empty acetabulum observed in subluxation become more prominent. The anterior and posterior limbus usually turn in the direction of the acetabulum. The acetabular aperture becomes narrow in the sagital plane and is pulled up superiorly, at times resembling a pointed arch.

The ligamentum teres often follows the migrating femoral head; acting as a retinaculum for the head it becomes elongated and hypertrophies. In many cases, however, it atrophies and ruptures, usually leaving remnants in the floor of the acetabulum and at its point of attachement to the head of the femur.

The superior limbus, which in subluxation of the head of the femur is pushed superiorly and pressed against the rim of the acetabulum, is now released from pressure. Sometimes it turns in the direction of the acetabulum. Occasionally it hypertrophies and may even form a proper "curtain" which covers the interior of the acetabulum. During reduction of the subluxation it acts as an undesirable interposition. Even in open reduction one can easily overlook this "curtain" of the limbus.

The depth of the acetabulum becomes considerably reduced. Various elements contribute to this. They include the inversion of the limbus, the enlargement of the pulvinar, the steep inclination of the acetabulum caused by pressure atrophy of the superior rim and finally the osseous bony condensation of the floor of the acetabulum.

b) The Rapidly Appearing Dislocation

The slowly progressing dislocation of the femoral head stands in contrast to the rapidly advancing full dislocation, i.e., the complete luxation. It may already occur in the embryonic stage where it is known as a teratogenic hip dislocation. It is usually accompanied by other congenital malformations. The teratogenic hip dislocation represents a specific problem and will not be discussed here.

The head of the femur may leave the acetabulum at any stage during the fetal period. The younger the fetus the more striking are the secondary deformities of the empty acetabulum. Conversely, the nearer the dislocation occurs to the perinatal period the better will be the condition of the acetabulum.

The fact that the head of the femur slips easily out of the acetabulum has the advantage that the biologically important acetabular lip is not exposed to long-lasting pressure and consequent atrophy. At operation, one finds even in marked dislocations of older children an unexpectedly deep acetabulum, after soft tissue accumulations have been removed surgically.

The clinical results are as follows: The acetabular deformities in teratogenic and early fetal subluxations and sabluxations are usually of such a severe nature that surgical intervention is required for their correction. The subluxations and dislocations originating in the perinatal period are in most cases amenable to conservative treatment. In older children even in these cases surgical measures are required.

IV. The Possibility of Formative Control of Acetabular Dysplasia

A peculiarity of the acetabulum is its susceptibility to being remodeled by exogenous factors. These may have a negative effect on the acetabulum. They are capable of transposing a normal condition to a dysplastic deformity; conversely, an existing dysplasia of the acetabulum may be caused to disappear.

Endogenous factors also play a role and act generally in a disturbing or inhibitory manner. The nature of these factors is difficult to comprehend. They may be hereditary (genetic factors), as well as the result of constitutional mesenchymal alterations. F. Becker considers their effects incalculable. Endogenous factors can very well have a negative influence on the treatment of the dysplastic hip, but do not cancel the effect of exogenous factors. For this reason, we shall direct our attention to exogenous factors whose effects are concrete and visible.

a) Acetabulum During Abduction Therapy

The efficacy of early treatment of hip dysplasia is based on its above-mentioned capability to respond to being molded. The formative element is the femur with its head whose proper seating in the acetabulum can produce reduction or even disappearance of the dysplasia phenomena.

The younger the child the greater the ability of the acetabulum to correct its deformity. The best age for abduction therapy is the first 9 months of the so-called extrauterine fetal period. Becker, Mittelmeier and other authors agree that a properly and deeply seated femoral head in the inferior part of the acetabulum is a precondition for self-restoration.

The upper part of the acetabulum and the acetabular lip must be absolutely free of pressure. Their growth must be unimpeded. The position of the femoral head deep in the acetabulum must be kept until the disturbed limbus unfolds itself again, until the contorted shape of the acetabulum regains its normal form, its upper margin forms a sharp angle. Osseous support for the femoral head from above is then assured.

Abduction therapy consists in progressively increasing abduction of the thighs in 90° of flexion until the Lorenz I position is reached. In this position the clinician will notice greater stability of the hips. However, there are certain risks in this position that one must be aware of. For example, in increased anteversion, the femoral head will press directly against the upper rim of the acetabulum, a fact to which Rohleder (cited by Mittelmeier) has called attention. Mittelmeier adds that in maximum abduction adverse pressure is exerted by the greater trochanter on the superior rim of the acetabulum and by the neck of the femur on the posterior acetabular rim, if internal rotation is not applied at the same time.

If abduction of the thigh in the Lorenz I position is excessive – i.e., hyper-abduction is present – then the femoral head is pressed forward, as P. Matzen has demonstrated with an antomic preparation. F. Becker, too, refers to this adverse lever action in the case of a poorly fitted abduction device.

The consequences of this anterior shift of the femoral head can be worse in cases where the anterior limbus is inverted, as is shown in Figure 7. The femoral head assumes an anterior position below the anterio-inferior spine of the ilium, forming a visible protrusion under Poupart's ligament in the groin. The forward displacement of the femoral head is equivalent to an anterior subluxation.

In these cases the anteriosuperior acetabular defect continues to exist after abduction therapy has been terminated. The joint is unstable. The imperfect position of the femoral head during abduction therapy leads to secondary deformities of the acetabulum. Redislocation, the inevitable result, can occur immediately after abduction treatment has been terminated, or even after a longer latency period.

We have operated on many patients with residual hip dislocations of this type and in every case found the dominant symptom to be a defect of the anteriosuperior acetabular rim with a steeply slanted acetabular roof. Since it usually affects 3–4-year-old children, we correct the acetabular defect surgically. Transiliac osteotomy with tilting of the upper half of the acetabulum is the procedure of choice.

Hypoflexion during abduction therapy is just as harmful as hyperabduction. If, as the result of a poorly fitted abduction device, abduction of the thigh is performed in less than 90° of flexion, the head of the femur will be centered in the superior quadrant of the acetabulum instead of in the inferior quadrant.

Cranial hyperflexion of the thigh favors better seating of the femoral head in the acetabulum. It is primarily useful in cases with increased anteversion of the femoral neck as well as in cases with pronounced hypotrophy of the anterior acetabular lip with a steeply slanted acetabulum.

b) Stabilization of the Femoral Head by Directional Osteotomies

As mentioned above, excessive anteversion of the femoral neck is an obstacle to proper stabilization of the hip. Increased valgus of the femoral neck has the same effect. These malpositions very often occur together. Both must be reduced by directional osteotomies, if physiologic values are exceeded, in the presence of a steeply slanted acetabular roof, and if there is no noticeable tendency to spontaneous correction.

The question arises as to what extent a derotation osteotomy alone may result in a spontaneous restoration of a steeply slanted acetabular roof.

The acetabular angle in newborns is normally about 30° and decreases during the first year of life to about 20°.

The acclivity of the acetabular roof remains unchanged during the second year of life. Only at the beginning of the third year does the upper part of the acetabulum begin to grow horizontally and to lengthen laterally.

The anterior acetabular rim gradually becomes sharp. According to J. Bedouelle, the superior acetabular angle becomes fully formed in the fourth year.

Therefore, one can only expect a directional osteotomy to be successful in producing spontaneous restitution of the upper part of the acetabulum up to the 3–4 years of life. If premature sclerosing of a steeply oblique acetabular roof is noted, it is usually a sign that the capacity for spontaneous restoration of the acetabular roof is exhausted. According to Hass (1951) this sclerosing is a more reliable index than a decrease in the C-E (Wiberg's) angle.

In children aged 4 or more with a high acetabular angle it is safer to combine directional osteotomy with surgical correction of the deficiency in the acetabular roof.

V. Factors Promoting Dysplasia

In general one can say that during the period of growth all factors leading to incorrect placement of the femoral head in the acetabulum can contribute to dysplasia of the acetabulum. They can be of kinetic or of static origins.

Functional deformities of the acetabulum in dislocated hips in patients with spina bifida and spastic paralysis are well known. In these cases periarticular muscular dysfunctions are the causative factors. The static-kinetic factors leading to deformity of the acetabulum may be intra- or extraarticular.

a) Intraarticular Factors

Decrease in volume of the acetabular cavity: Physiologic structures of the acetabulum, such as the ligamentum teres and the fat pad, may hypertrophy under pathologic conditions and displace the femoral head laterally. Usually they are secondary findings accompanying dislocations of the hip. They are associated with capsular folds within the acetabulum and with superior displacement of the transverse ligament resulting from tension of the ligamentum teres if it is not torn by the migration of the acetabular head. These pathologic soft tissue changes of the inferior sector of the acetabulum, as well as the above-mentioned hypertrophy of the inferiorly inverted limbus in the cranial sector resist every attempt to position the femoral head correctly in the acetabulum, be it via a directional osteotomy or an acetabuloplasty with or without tilting of the entire acetabulum.

Interpostions of these structures must be eliminated surgically while taking care to preserve the true fat pad. Soft tissue hypertrophy usually is less pronounced on the fat pads themselves than on the remaining surrounding structures. Leaving the fat pads is of value for the function of the reduced head of the femur. Removal of the soft tissue alone, though, is insufficient if bony condensation of the floor of the acetabulum and flattening of the rims is also present.

b) Persistent Increased Anteversion of the Femoral Neck

The high degree of anteversion in the newborn decreases with the growth of the child, usually in the second year of life. This reduction coincides with the growth of the acetabular lip and with the increase in the acetabular angle. If for any reason increased anteversion persists, the hip joint may be threatend by instability which – as mentioned above – may be acute or chronic.

During abduction therapy, especially if it was begun relatively late, one can often notice that the hip is stable in abduction and internal rotation. However, there is an immediate loss of stability when the limb is placed in an ambulatory position and the hip reluxates. The cause for this is the increased anteversion.

We have seen failures after simple surgical reduction, even in infants. In spite of surgically correct repositioning of the femoral head in the acetabulum we had encountered redislocations in cases where the increased anteversion went untreated. It is therefore advisable in every surgical reduction to test the stability of the hip *not* in abduction but with the limb in the neutral ambulatory position.

The question now remains how far the acetabulum is able to reduce the amount of anteversion. Although spontaneous reduction of acetabular dysplasia together with a decrease in the angle of anteversion is observed in infants, every case of increased femoral neck anteversion should be carefully followed. Roentgenograms taken in the Rippstein position help to clarify the situation. The question of the influence of the acetabulum on anteversion of the neck of the femur will be dealt with further in the discussion of surgical procedures.

c) Increased Valgus of the Neck of the Femur

High valgus angles of the femoral neck are often seen after excessively prolonged periods of abduction therapy. If the acetabulum has already developed a sharp angle and is, on the whole, well formed, the valgus position may reduce spontaneously.

However, if there is a tendency to lateral displacement of the capital femoral epiphysis relative to the neck of the femur or if the valgus position of the femoral neck is combined with increased anteversion, the danger of a secondary acetabular deformity is great. A well-timed derotation osteotomy is indicated.

d) Malpositions of the Pelvis

A horizontal tilt of the pelvis places the acetabula on unequal levels. The result is that in the position of gait the leg with the lower acetabulum is in abduction while the contralateral leg is in adduction. Lasting adduction has an adverse effect on an acetabulum predisposed to dysplasia. Diminution of the contact surface between the acetabulum and femoral head causes pressure to be concentrated on the upper part of the acetabulum with familiar results. The most frequent causes of horizontal pelvic tilt are low lumbar scoliosis and discrepancies in leg length.

1. Low Lumbosacral Scoliosis

An example will clearly illustrate the consequences of a long-standing pelvic tilt:

A female (A. L. 12607) received abduction therapy to correct bilateral dislocation of the hips several weeks after her birth (Fig. 8a). Nevertheless, trouble arose in applying an abduction device because of a marked pelvic tilt, the result of congenital lumbosacral scoliosis with spina bifida. After 4 months, only the more caudal hip had been reduced (Fig. 8b). The other hip had to be reduced surgically. At the age of 19 months Salter's innominate osteotomy, as modified by us, was carried out. Approximately 2-cm-thick cancellous bone cubes of lyophilized homologous bone were placed in the osteotomy gap, not only to increase the acetabular angle but to position the acetabulum more caudal and thus achieve a better horizontal position of both hips (Fig. 8d). One year later, the roentgenogram (Fig. 8c) shows a completely reconstructed ilium. The ipsilateral head of the femur has been reduced with slight lateralization. The contralateral hip was completely normal. After another year – the child was then $4^1/_2$ years old – the roentgenogram shows a good reposition (Fig. 8e). The valgus position of the right femoral neck has increased, the plate of the capital femoral epiphyses is placed horizontally, and an

a b c

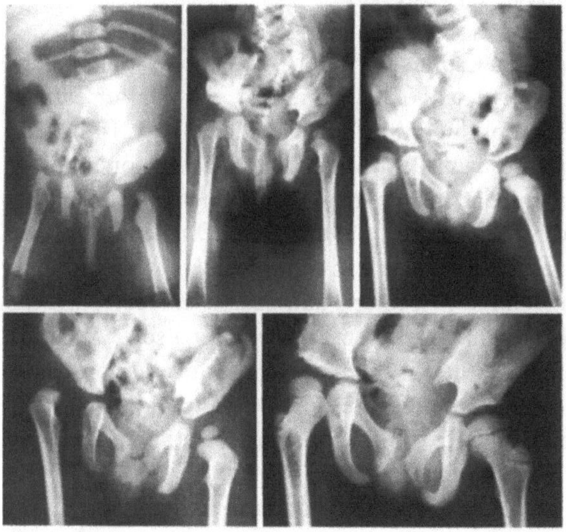

d e

Fig. 8a–e. (a) A. L. 12607. Girl, 5 months old, with extreme congenital lumbosacral scoliosis with spina bifida and pelvic tilt. Bilateral hip dislocation. (b) Four months after abduction therapy. Left-sided *d* reduction only. (d) Two months after Salter's osteotomy with large lyophilized bone wedges to obtain horizontal placement of the acetabulum. (c) One year after operation. (e) Two years after operation. Pelvic tilt continues to compromise the right hip joint despite reduction. Osteotomy of spinal column impossible because of coexisting congenital kidney defect

additional valgus position of the epiphysis relative to the neck of the femur is noted. Clinically the result is good. Gait is normal. The extreme scoliosis remains. The circumstances of this case call for an osteotomy to eliminate the lumbosacral scoliosis. This, hoever, was impossible, because of the coexistence of a horseshoe kidney with renal insufficiency.

2. Unequal Leg Length

Discrepancies in leg length may result from shortening or lengthening of a lower limb. In the treatment of hip dislocations, the usual causes of leg length discrepancies are unilateral dislocation or subluxation, unilateral coxa vara or coxa valga, or unilateral genu valgum. In addition, deliberate surgical shortening of the femoral shaft as well as postoperative growth stimuli (e.g., intertrochanteric osteotomy) may be responsible for disproportionate leg lengths.

Discrepancies in leg length produce a pelvic tilt with the consequences mentioned above. Often, discrepancies occurring during treatment of hip dysplasias are noticed too late or are even overlooked. In most cases one is dealing with a bilateral dysplasia in which one hip is considered to be healed. The well-known problem of the so-called normal hip often has its origin in a leg length discrepancy. On the other hand, one can obtain better conditions for healing by lengthening the contralateral leg functionally with the use of a lift in the shoe in a slightly dysplastic acetabulum, e.g., following surgical reconstruction.

C. Persistent Dysplasia of the Acetabulum

Clinical experience demonstrates that sooner or later every hip dysplasia leads to osteoarthrosis with its well-known sequelae. Therefore, the goal of earliest treatment is to remodel the dysplastic hip joint into one that is normal anatomically and functionally. To what extent endogenous factors inhibit, disturb, and otherwise influence the end results remains an open question.

Surgical treatment of hip dysplasia has the same goal. One endeavors to obtain the most complete normalization of the dysplastic joint with the least possible intervention. In small children it often suffices to correct only the primary defect. Thereafter, the secondary defect will correct itself. Accurate recognition of the primary defect by the surgeon and proper evaluation of the existing potential for spontaneous correction are decisive. The older the child and the more extensive the hip dysplasia, the more complicated and extensive will be the surgical reconstructive intervention.

Surgery must be performed with care and should not damage the blood supply and cartilaginous growth zones of the hip. The blood supply for the acetabulum, which I will not describe in detail, is generally less endangered by approaches at the acetabulum than at the coxal end of the femur.

With respect to growth zones, one should mention the triradiate cartilage, which joins the ilium, ischium, and pubis, the cartilaginous part of the acetabular lip and the cartilaginous lining of the cavity which acts as growing epiphyseal cartilage. Between the 7th and 9th years of life, bony deposits (ossa cotyloidea) appear in various parts of the acetabulum (Fig. 9). At age 15 fusion begins and this process is completed at age 18–20 (according to Perna, Pratje; cited by A. Santacroce).

There are numerous methods of surgical treatment of hip dysplasia. I shall limit my discussion to those procedures with which I am personally familiar.

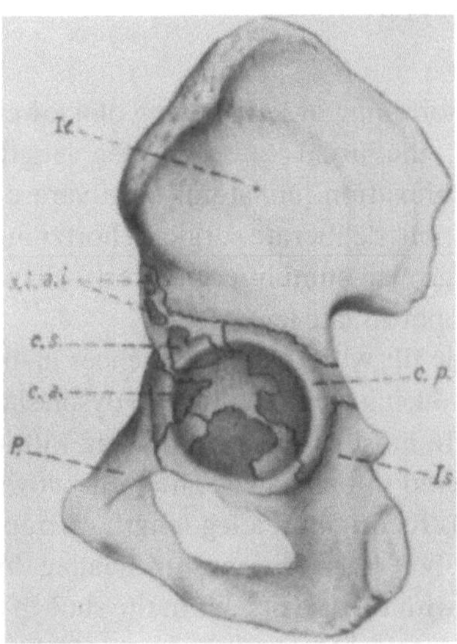

Fig. 9 *Ie s.i.a.i.* Anterior iliac spine. *c.s.* Superior cotyloid. *c.a.* Anterior cotyloid. *P* Pubic bone. *c.p.* Posterior cotyloid. *Is* Ischium. (From Santacroce, A.: Trattamento chirurgico della sublussazione cong. dell'anca. Proc. 49th Congr. Soc. Ital. Orthop. and Trauma., Venice 1946, p. 16)

a) Acetabular Roof Shelf Arthroplasty

Years ago (ca. 1920 and later) reconstruction of the acetabular roof was considered to be the treatment of choice for correcting an acetabular defect. The acetabular roof, formed of bone grafts, was expected to act as an abutment for the femoral head. At that time, acetabular roof "plasties" were new and marked a great advance in the surgical treatment of congenital dysplasia.

Nowadays, the indications for this operation are limited. However, when indicated, it can still produce good results. I have performed acetabular roof "plasties" since 1927 and would like to draw attention to a phenomenon that is sometimes forgotten: namely the biologic effect of bone grafts on the formation of the acetabulum.

In 1932, I presented two cases of subluxation in children aged 5 and 7. I performed a semicircular supraacetabular deep osteotomy and by turning the upper half of the acetabulum, including the femoral head, inferiorly obtained a stable seating of the femoral head. Bone grafts taken from the tibia were placed into the osteotomy space.

Roentgen pictures show the reposition of the femoral head. However, the tibial bone grafts were placed much too high to actually act as an abutment for the femoral head. In spite of this, within 39 months an acetabular lip formed which adequately covered the femoral head (Fig. 10a, b). The action of the bone grafts was not mechanical but rather biologic in that they stimulated the growth potential within the acetabular lip. This observation was the starting point for developing a procedure which I later named transiliac osteotomy.

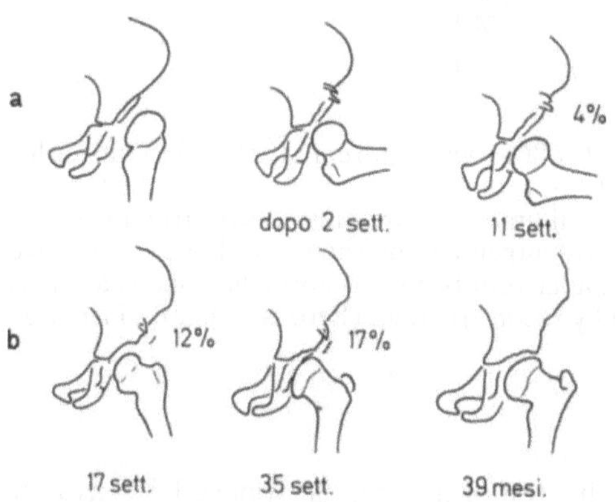

Fig. 10. Girl of 5 years with congenital subluxation. Open reduction with semicircular supra-acetabular osteotomy and plastic surgery of the acetabular roof. Result after 2–35 weeks and 39 months

Stracker and especially Hauberg were justified in advocating early reconstruction of the acetabular roof. I have employed the shelf acetabular roof arthroplasty as an additional measure in surgical reduction of the hip (Fig. 11, a–d). Its biologic effect can, of course, only be expected in infants. In older children and adults, reconstruction of the acetabular roof can only play a supplementary mechanical role, i.e., extending the missing supporting surface of the acetabulum, but only after or while undertaking reconstruction of the statics and kinetics of the dysplastic hip joint.

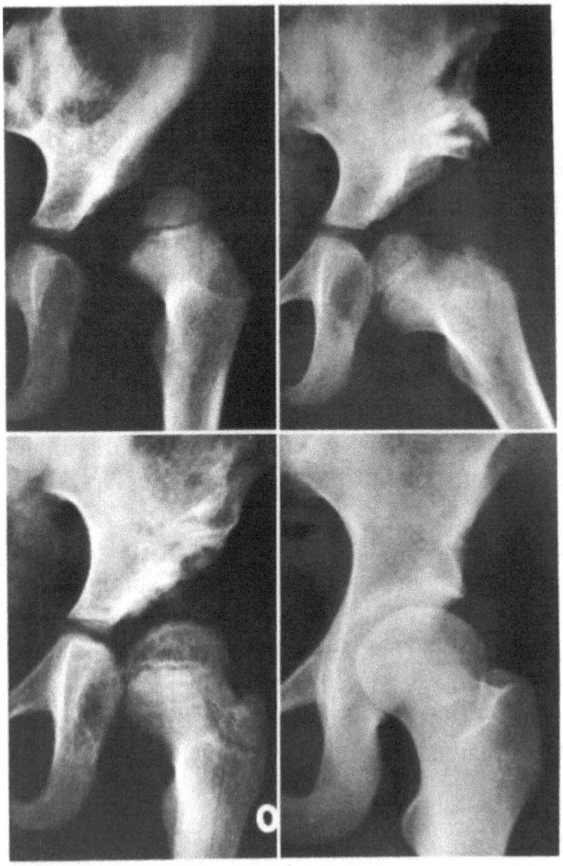

Fig. 11a–d. (a) Four-year-old girl (W. W. 6869) with untreated left-sided hip dislocation. (b) After exposing the joint capsule – without opening the joint – the femoral head is seated in the original acetabulum by thumb pressure only. Reconstruction of the acetabular roof completes the operation. Roentgenograms show that bone grafts have been placed much too high. (c) The acetabular roof begins to normalize one year later. (d) After 13 years the acetabular lip is fully reconstructed. There is a slightly increased valgus of the femoral neck

Following acetabular roof plasty the femoral head is opposed by hyaline cartilage only in the acetabulum. The rest is covered by the bone graft. Only the capsule separates the femoral head from the upper roof of the acetabulum. The wider the contact surface with the cartilaginous part of the acetabulum, the smaller will be the bony area of the acetabular roof, which does not possess any cartilage.

Although satisfactory results of some acetabular roof plasties persist for years into adulthood, it is advisable in such operations to extend the cartilaginous part of the abutment as wide as possible by means of a simultaneous rotation osteotomy.

b) Colonna's Capsular Acetabuloplasty

There are dislocated hips in which disproportions between the shape of the acetabulum and the size and form of the femoral head make it difficult to reduce and maintain the femoral head in proper position. Colonna has developed a sound method to eliminate these difficulties by shaping the acetabulum by curetting the cavity. The femoral head together with its enclosing capsule is then replaced in the joint where it is protected from direct contact with the surgically denuded interior of the cavity by the capsule.

The concept of this method was convincing, but long-term results have not met our expectations, as has been confirmed by A. N. Witt among others. Colonna has not published any statistical studies of his results. The main reason for the disappointing results was the pressing of the femoral head against the roof of the acetabulum, exerted by the pelvifemoral muscles which were displaced during dislocation. We have modified Colonna's operation by attempting to eliminate this damaging pressure through shortening the length of the femoral shaft. In the years 1953–1967, 1274 hips were treated in our clinic according to this method. The results were reported in Vienna in 1969.

In this paper only the effects of the procedure on the acetabulum will be described. The shaping and deepening of the acetabular cavity can only be done at the expense of the acetabular cartilage. The question arises as to what effect the removal of cartilage from the acetabulum and above all from the Y line and from the acetabular lip has on the further growth of the acetabulum.

The interesting descriptions of P. Otte (1969) have contributed much to our understanding of these growth processes. According to Otte the growth activity of the triradiate cartilage is bipolar, transverse and synchronous with the general alteration taking place in the growing pelvis of the child. Theoretically, complete absence of the growth capability of the triradiate cartilage would be followed by a cessation of growth of the acetabulum cranially, as well as by rarefaction of the floor of the acetabulum. Cessation of the activity of the acetabular lip would end the lateral growth of the superior acetabular rim. Bernbeck calls this area the "nucleus of the acetabulum" *(Pfannenkern),* the site where periosteal and perichondral ossification are joined. It is here that the repair of the acetabular roof take place.

Postoperatively, further development of the acetabulum therefore depends on the type and severity of surgical injury to the cartilagious elements. In the surgical remodeling of the acetabulum according to Colonna we were always careful to preserve the acetabular nucleus. This growth zone must be viewed as an area that must be protected with utmost care. For this reason it is important to identify the position of the triradiate cartilage in the original acetabulum at the beginning of the operation in order that the curetting is not unnecessarily excessive. If at all possible, the hollowing out of the acetabular roof must be done below the upper rim of the original acetabulum. It is sometimes enough to remove only one layer from the cartilaginous lining for adequate refashioning of the acetabulum. In our experience the remaining cartilaginous lining preserves its growth viability. There is agreement as to the relatively good results obtained with this procedure in children less than 5 years of age as opposed to the much worse results reported in older children.

The femoral head, of course, has an important influence on the further restructuring of the acetabulum. We have tried to normalize its influence by suitable derotation osteotomies of the femoral neck and by shortening the length of the femoral shaft. These corrections are done at the same time as the reduction of the femoral head. In high dislocations where the length of the shaft had not been shortened enough one can observe a gradual cranial migration of the femoral head in the acetabulum.

Enlarging the acetabular cavity by curettage induces secondary reactions in almost all cases. They appear in many variations, depending on the type and localization of the surgical lesion of the cartilage as well as on the age of the child. The most frequent reactions are sclerosis and a certain indistinctness of the acetabular rims. Very often the bony floor of the acetabulum becomes thickened (thick "teardrop"). On the other hand, the acetabular floor may at times rarefy with protrusion in the direction of the pelvis. Occasionally growth of both halves of the acetabulum – superior and inferior – was greater than in the healthy contralateral acetabulum in the presence of a partially preserved Y line. In those cases the acetabulum became larger. If this was associated with a thickening of the acetabular floor, the acetabulum in time became shallower. I have observed in many acetabula a greater increase in growth in the inferior section, in others only in its superior part. Enlargement of the superior section of the acetabulum is usually accompanied by a widening of the acetabular lip through lateral expansion. By this means, the acetabulum becomes deeper.

If there is considerable damage to the Y line, it ossifies prematurely. The acetabulum becomes smaller and the femoral head seated in it also becomes smaller than the femoral head of the contralateral side. Irregular growth of the halves of the acetabulum produces distortion of its contours. If the entire acetabular cartilage is removed, as is the case in older children, the femoral head faces unprotected bone tissue with only a layer of joint capsule interposed. This is probably the main reason why even the best early results develop prearthrotic changes between 20 and 30 years of age. Although the capsular head is transformed into a cartilage-like tissue – as our microscopic studies have demonstrated – it is no substitute for the biologically valuable hyaline cartilage.

Capsular acetabulopasty provides a particular opportunity to study the pathophysiology of the growing acetabulum. We have initiated such investigations. Nowadays, capsular acetabuloplasty is very limited in its indications. Other, more recent procedures give better results.

c) Salter's Innominate Osteotomy

Salter proceeded on the assumption that in dysplastic hips the acetabulum as a whole is falsely positioned in the pelvis. The plane of its aperture is too steeply slanted and turned too far laterally. Salter tilts the entire acetabulum with its contents anteriorly and inferiorly over the femoral head whereby he obtains a good abutment lined with hyaline cartilage. The symphysis pubis is used as the hinge.

The osteotomy is performed above the protecting osteochondral area of the acetabular lip. Therefore, neither this growth zone nor the triradiate cartilage is damaged, which is an advantage of the operation. The drawbacks of Salter's procedure are judged to be the following: The inferiorly shifted acetabulum produces a functional elongation of the ipsilateral leg and a pelvic tilt in the standing position (Mittelmeier). The wedge-shaped bone graft, which ensures the tilt of the acetabulum, places the superior part of the acetabulum under continuous pressure against the femoral head (Hoffmann-Daimler). The inferior displacement is opposed by the gluteal muscles and the adductors; on this account Morscher recommends that a derotation osteotomy be carried out at the same time. Salter feels that a myotomy of the adductors is sufficient.

G. Thomas criticizes the flattening of the posterior rim.

The horizontal level of the plane of the pelvic inlet rotates in such a way that the posterior acetabular rim is displaced superiorly while the superior rim is displaced anteriorly. The anteroposterior roentgenogram clearly demonstrates the lowering of the superior acetabular rim but is deceptive in regard to the posterior rim. Special films, as suggested by Goeb, are indicated.

In extreme acetabular acclivity, one does not obtain a sufficient acetabular tilt (Mittelmeier). This also holds true for acetabula of older children in whom the symphysis is less flexible. In vertically ovoid acetabula the transposition of the acetabulum results in an incongruence of the joint (Mittelmeier). In addition, the lateral displacement of the femoral head does not usually correct itself spontaneously in Salter's procedure (Morscher).

Since we already had years of experience with our transiliac osteotomy, we soon departed from Salter's original operation, using it when necessary in combination with supplementary procedures which met all the above mentioned requirements. These were as follows: in lateral displacement of the femoral head: arthrotomy with excision of the interposed structures (limbus, transverse ligament, hypertrophied ligamentum teres, etc.); in malposition of the femoral neck: derotation osteotomies; performing at the same time, if necessary, shortening of the femoral shaft in dislocations. Using these procedures in small children we have observed acetabula which assumed an almost normal shape within 2–3 years.

The inferior dislocation of the acetabulum following an operation employing larger bone grafts is corrected within a few years. The innominate osteotomy with a wedge-shaped bone graft, even if lyophilized bone is used, has definite stimulatory effect on the acetabular lip and femoral head in small children. This is clearly demonstrated on a roentgenogram by comparison to the contralateral side. In some cases almost no signs of the operation can be noted in the roentgenogram after several years.

Although Salter's osteotomy was a great step forward in the surgical treatment of hip dysplasia we have reverted to our transiliac osteotomy, which not only produces results as good as Salter's procedure but is much simpler and safer. We have thus markedly limited the indication for Salter's operation.

d) Transiliac Osteotomy

As mentioned above in the discussion of acetabular roof shelf arthroplasty, it was in 1929 and 1930 that we began to develop our procedure of rotating the upper half of the steeply slanted acetabulum. My first results were published in 1931. The procedures of Spitzy and Lance served as my point of departure.

The considerable increase in our knowledge of the pathology of hip dysplasia in recent years has led to new technical refinements in these surgical procedures. Since 1958 I have called the operation "supraacetabular and transiliac osteotomy." The procedure resembles – but not entirely – Pemberton's and also the one carried out in recent years by Mittelmeier. I shall not go into the technical details of the operation, but will confine myself to a discussion of the development of the shape of the acetabulum which is achieved by this procedure.

The osteotomy is carried out lower than in Salter's procedure, which not only transsects the lateral cortical substance of the innominate bone but also the medial one. It does not extend to the triradiate cartilage, as suggested by Pemberton, and may – but need not always – divide the corticalis in the sciatic notch, as in Salter's operation. For fixation of the deflected lamella of the acetabular roof, bone grafts are taken from the neighboring upper part of the ilium or else a wedge of bone from the femur is used. In small children, who have a very thin ilium, we use lyophilized homogeneous wedges of cancellous bone, which heal very well albeit somewhat more slowly.

On no account should the osteochondral zone of the acetabular lip be damaged, but the deflected lamella of the acetabular roof should not be too thick. It must be flexible enough to allow sufficient tilting of the damaged superior-anterior rim downward and the posterior rim forward. Both cortical walls must be sufficiently incised to permit shaping of the acetabular roof lamella as desired.

The transiliac osteotomy – like Salter's osteotomy – does not harm the growth centers of the acetabulum and the femoral head retains its protective covering of hyaline cartilage. In most cases the transiliac osteotomy is carried out in combination with other corrective procedures, as is our practice with Salter's osteotomy. In extreme coxa valga with a slanting acetabulum we often find a large inverted eniscus-like limbus interposed between the femoral head and acetabular roof, producing an intraarticular incongruence. In all cases where interposition is suspected, an arthrotomy should be done. A derotation osteotomy carried out at the same time will provide correct centering of the femoral neck axis. Any intraarticular compression, as seen in high subluxations and in dislocations, are carefully eliminated by shortening the length of the femoral shaft. According to this concept, up to now we have obtained the best results in comparison to other methods.

The age of the child is also decisive. In children over 6 or 7 years the lamella of the acetabular roof is not pliant enough to be turned down and made to conform to the femoral head. In addition the biologically stimulative effect of the bone grafts is lessened. In no cases have we observed trophic disturbances in the region of the deflected lamella of the acetabular roof.

The postoperative secondary stimulatory effects are almost the same as those following Salter's osteotomy. Hypertrophy of the superior acetabulum resulting from intensive lateral growth of the acetabular lip, and enlargement of the femoral head are observed. Secondary bony condensation of the acetabular floor is rare. Changes in the area of the triradiate cartilage have not been noted.

e) Chiari's Pelvic Osteotomy

Chiari's pelvic osteotomy creates immediate support for the femoral head from above provided that the osteotomy is carried out in a line running through the cancellous substance of the innominate bone above the original acetabulum. The more proximal the line of the osteotomy, the narrower is the supportive surface. This is due to the normal anatomic thinness of the upper part of the ilium. At times the cancellous bone mass may also become narrow as the result of a deep secondary acetabulum that has formed in the anterior rim in cases of subluxation. In this situation the supportive surface will be disproportionate to the size of the femoral head. If such narrow supporting surfaces are present, they will result in deficient coverage of the remodeled acetabulum.

As an operation designed to fashion an acetabulum, Chiari's osteotomy is said to have several disadvantages: The new acetabular roof is flat instead of round and does not conform to the spherical form of the femoral head. In our experience, after several months a vault is formed in the flat roof of the acetabulum through the functional activities of the femoral head. The cancellous bone tissue of the roof proves to be sufficiently responsive. Very often the femoral head migrates slightly cranially, which, has the effect of shortening the length of the leg.

A. N. Witt calls attention to the increased acetabular acclivity following pelvic osteotomy which is caused by the medial displacement of the acetabular fragments. The hyaline supportive surface for the femoral head, which is small in any case, is diminished even further, and the steeply slanted acetabulum permits migration of the femoral head superiorly. A further disadvantage of the pelvic osteotomy of Chiari is that the femoral head faces raw bone.

In the opinion of most authors the joint capsule, although it covers the femoral head, is no satisfactory substitute for the biological properties of hyaline cartilage. Therefore it is Hackenbroch's opinion that this must result in the development of early prearthroses. Our material appears to confirm this.

In regard to the capsular covering of the femoral head, the results from Chiari's osteotomy are quite similar to those of Colonna's capsular acetabuloplasty. The danger of prearthrosis is greater when the femoral neck is malpositioned (e.g., in marked valgus) and when the newly fashioned acetabulum does not conform adequately to the femoral head, which results in an area of poorly distributed weight-bearing. A properly timed rotation osteotomy is indicated in such cases. For this reason, H. Wagner attempts to enlarge the hyaline covering by means of his spherical acetabular osteotomy. The objection that the medially shifted acetabulum narrows the minor pelvis and thus forms an obstacle to subsequent labor of childbirth has been refuted by Chiari.

Our roentgenologic observations confirm this. The plane of the pelvic inlet – even when markedly narrowed – usually broadens with the passage of years and becomes almost normal. The great plasticity of the growing pelvis is often capable of compensating for even large surgical errors. After years an adequate weight-bearing acetabulum can be formed in spite of total slippage of the acetabular fragments medially. The same can be said for the steplike acetabular roof. This occurs if the osteotomy is carried out above the level of the superior acetabular rim. Even this unevenness in the arch of the acetabular roof can smooth out in time.

The fault most difficult to eliminate after osteotomy is posterior slipping of the acetabular fragments. The hip joint on the operated side will be situated posterior to the horizontal plane of the contralateral hip, if this displacement is not corrected. This displacement is difficult to visualize in the anteroposterior roentgenogram, but is often the reason for subsequently poor functional late results despite an apparently good roentgen appearance.

Fixation of the fragments during operation is definitely indicated as posterior displacement often happens in a postoperative plaster cast. The acetabulum as fashioned according to Chiari requires months and sometimes years before it is finally reconstructed. Weight-bearing must not be attempted too early, and the early results should not be regarded as end results. The more carefully and correctly the acetabulum is shaped, the earlier and better will be the final outcome.

In older children, Chiari's pelvic osteotomy is sometimes the only procedure of choice. It is, however, rarely indicated in younger children.

A review of the procedures employed for reshaping the acetabulum demonstrates that poor as well as good results can be expected. Even the best early reults may, after years, worsen because of premature articular degeneration. Very frequently these are joints which were damaged by previous treatment. The genetic factor can play a decisive role here. Its cause may be a constitutional mesenchymal inferiority.

Nevertheless, the surgeon is justified in his attempt at functional improvement of a defective hip joint. The goal of treatment, as A. N. Witt so well puts it, is to "secure for the person affected – in most cases a girl – in the most active time of her life, a practically normal life with an inconspicuous gait."

The frequently very good results which can be achieved with radial measures to reshape the acetabulum do not release the orthopaedic surgeon from his duty to use conservative methods in early treatment and, if these fail, from his duty to operate early in young children when the plasticity of the hip joint is optimal, therefore contributing to good results.

References

Becker, F.: Z. Orthop. **106,** 1 (1968)
Becker, F.: Z. Orthop. **95,** 2 (1961)
Becker, F.: Arch. orthop. Unfall-Chir. **55,** (1963)
Bedouelle, J.: Rev. Orthop. **40,** 5–6 (1954)
Bernbeck, R.: Kinderorthopädie. Stuttgart: G. Thieme 1954
Bernbeck, R.: Verh. d. Deutsch. Ges. f. Orth. u. Traumat. 56. Kongreß, Wien 1969, S. 131–132 Stuttgart: F. Enke 1970
Bernbeck, R.: Verh. d. Deutsch. Ges. f. Orthop. u. Traumat. 56. Kongreß, Wien 1969, S. 131. Stuttgart: F. Enke 1970
Büschelberger, H. Beitr. Orthop. Traum. **11,** 535 (1964)
Chandler, Bone surg. **XI,** 3 (1929)
Chapchal, G.: Verh. d. Deutsch. Ges. f. Orth. u. Traumat. 56. Kongreß, Wien 1969, S. 217 Stuttgart: F. Enke
Chiari, K.: Wien. med. Wschr. **38,** 1953
Chiari, K.: Bericht über die Beckenosteotomie als Pfannendachplastik nach eigener Methode. In: Chapchal, G.: Beckenosteotomie – Pfannendachplastik, S. 70–75. Stuttgart: G. Thieme 1965
Chiari, K.: Der pfannenbildende Eingriff. Verh. d. Deutsch. Ges. f. Orthop. u. Traumat. Wien 1969, S. 193–201. Stuttgart: F. Enke 1970
Colonna, P. C.: Surg. Gynec. Obstet. **63,** 777–784 (1936)
Colonna, P. C.: J. Bone **35 A,** 179–197 (1953)
Colonna, P. C.: J. Bone Surg. **47–A,** 437–449 (1965)
Le Damany, P.: La luxation congenitale de la hanche. Paris: Felix Alcan. 1912 und Paris: Ernst Famanion 1923
Dega, W.: Chir. Narzad. Ruchu **I,** 4 (1929)
Dega, W.: Now. lek. **3,** (1930)
Dega, W.: Chir. Narzad. Ruchu **V,** 11 (1932)
Dega, W.: Chir. Organi Mov. **XVIII,** 5 (1933)
Dega, W.: Prophylaxie, depistage précoce et traitement immédiat de la dysplasie cong. de la hanche. Centre Internat. Infance. Réunions et Conférences VII. Paris 1960
Dega, W.: Contributo allo studio clinico della riconstruzione del tetto cotiloideo. Atti del XXIII. Congresso della Soc. Italiana di Ortopedia. Bologna 15–17, X, 1932
Dega, W.: La prophylaxie de la luxation cong. de la hance chez les nouveau-nés. VII Congr. de la Soc. Internat. de Chir. Orthop. et de Traumat. Barcelone 16–21, IX, 1957
Dega, W.: Chir. Nazad. Ruchu **IV,** 533–594 (1931)
Dega, W.: Chir. Narzad, Ruchu **VI,** 721–733 (1933)
Dega, W.: Pol. Med. Hist. and Science Bull. **II,** 3–4 (1959)
Dega, W.: J. Bone Surg. **41–A,** 5 (1959)
Dega, W.: Beitr. Orthop. Traum. **II,** 642 (1964)
Dega, W.: Der klinische Wert der Pfannendachplastik in der Behandlung d. angeb. Hüftluxation. In: Chapchal, G.: Beckenosteotomie – Pfannendachplastik. Stuttgart: G. Thieme 1965
Dega, W.: Arch. orthop. Unfall-Chir. **60,** 16–29 (1966)
Dega, W.: Hüftreposition mit Rekonstruktion der anatomischen Gelenkform nach Colonna, Zahradnicek u. a. und die abstützenden Osteotomien. Verh. d. Deutsch. Ges. f. Orthop. u. Traumat. 56. Kongreß, Wien 1969
Goeb: zitiert nach H. Thomas
Graf, P.: Zur Lehre von d. Entstehung d. angeb. Hüftverrenkung. Brun's Beitr. klin. Chir. **64,** (1909)
Hackenbroch, H.: Die Pfannendachplastik und die Beckenosteotomie und die varisierende derotierende Osteotomie im Lichte der Präarthrose. In: Chapchal, G.: Beckenosteotomie – Pfannendachplastik, S. 1–6. Stuttgart: G. Thieme 1965
Harrenstein, R. J.: Z. orthop. Chir. **49,** (1928)
Hauberg, G.: Die Frühpfannendachplastik. In: Chapchal, G.: Beckenosteotomie-Pfannendachplastik, S. 30–31. Stuttgart: G. Thieme 1965
Hass, J.: Congenital Dislocation of the Hip. Charles. Springfield, Illinois: C. Thomas. 1951

Hoffmann-Daimler, S.: Beitr. Orthop. Traum. **9,** 1967
Hoffmann-Daimler, S.: Verh. d. Deutsch. Ges. f. Orthop. u. Traumat. 56. Kongreß, Wien 1969, S. 210–212. Stuttgart: F. Enke 1970
Lance, M.: Presse méd. **56,** (1925)
Matzen, P. E.: Lehrbuch der Orthopädie. Berlin: VEB Verlag Volk. u. Gesundheit 1967
Mittelmeier, H.: Beckenosteotomie – Pfannendachplastik im Kleinkindesalter. In: Chapchal, G.: Beckenosteotomie, Pfannendachplastik, S. 64–65. Stuttgart: G. Thieme 1965
Mittelmeier, H.: Arch. orthop. Unfall-Chir. **52,** (1961)
Morscher, E.: Kombinierte Beckenosteotomie nach Salter mit varisierender Detorsionsosteotomie am oberen Femurenende. In: Chapchal, G.: Beckenosteotomie – Pfannendachplastik, S. 78–87. Stuttgart: G. Thieme 1965
Ortolani, M.: Rev. Chir. Orthop. **44,** 1 (1958)
Otte, P.: Zur Pfannendachentwicklung des Hüftgelenks. Verh. d. deutsch. Ges. f. Orth. u. Traum. 56. Kongreß, Wien 17–20. IX. 1969, S. 63–75. Stuttgart: F. Enke 1970
Pemberton P. A.: J. Bone Surg. **40–A** (1958)
Pemberton P. A.: J. Bone Surg. **47–A,** 65 (1965) (typ script 1961)
Retting, H.: Erfahrungen mit der osteotomia innominata (Salter). In: Chapchal, G.: Beckenosteotomie / Pfannendachplastik, S. 104–105. Stuttgart: G. Thieme 1965
Salter, R. B.: J. Bone J. Surg. 518–539 (1961)
Salter, R. B.: J. Bone J. Surg. **43–B,** 518 (1965)
Santacroce, A.: Relazione al 49 Congresso della Soc. Italiana di Ortopedia e di Traumatologia, S. 19–22. Venezia: 1964
Stracker, A. O.: Frühzeitige Pfannendachplastik bei Hüftdysplasie. Z. Orthop. **95,** (1960)
Thomas G.: Zur operativen Technik der Pfannendachplastik. In: Chapchal, G.: Beckenosteotomie – Pfannendachplastik, S. 40–42, 125. Stuttgart: G. Thieme: 1965
Tönnis, D.: Über die Änderungen des Pfannendachwinkels der Hüftgelenke bei Dreh- und Kippstellungen des kindlichen Beckens. Z. Orthop. **96,** 462 (1962)
Wagner, H.: Korrektur der Hüftgelenksdysplasie durch die sphärische Pfannendachplastik. In: Chapchal, G.: Beckenosteotomie und Pfannendachplastik, S. 68–69. Stuttgart: G. Thieme 1965
Wiberg, G.: J. Bone J. Surg. **35–A,** 65 (1953)
Witt, A. N.: Verh. d. Deutsch. Ges. f. Orthop. u. Traumat. 56. Kongreß, Wien. 1969, S. 192. Stuttgart: F. Enke 1970

English translation from the German edition *Der Orthopäde,* Vol. 2, pp. 202–218 (1973),

Radiologic Interpretation of Dysplasia of the Acetabulum

W. Schuster*

In our pediatric case material, about 10% of all radiologic examinations during infancy comprise standard pelvic X-rays. In 1972, 604 pelvic X-rays of infants less than 1 year old were taken at the Children's Hospital of the University of Erlangen-Nürnberg to determine the presence of dysplasia or dislocation of the hip.

Since so-called congenital dislocation of the hip develops as a result of a connatal dysplasia of the entire hip-joint area, dysplasia of the acetabulum assumes a specific significance.

True congenital dislocation of the hip occurs only among 2%–4% of all newborn infants, then usually in conjunction with other malformations (Fig. 1). In most cases, dislocation develops during the first year of life and arises from dysplasia of the acetabulum. The incidence of dysplasia of the hip-joint of newborns has been variously reported in the literature by estimates that fluctuate from 1%–10%. We have calculated that in about 8000 pediatric examinations of newborns at the Women's Hospital of the University of Erlangen-Nürnberg during the past 4 years, 5% of the infants had positive Ortolani signs. We were able to establish a preponderance in females at a ratio of 6:1, as

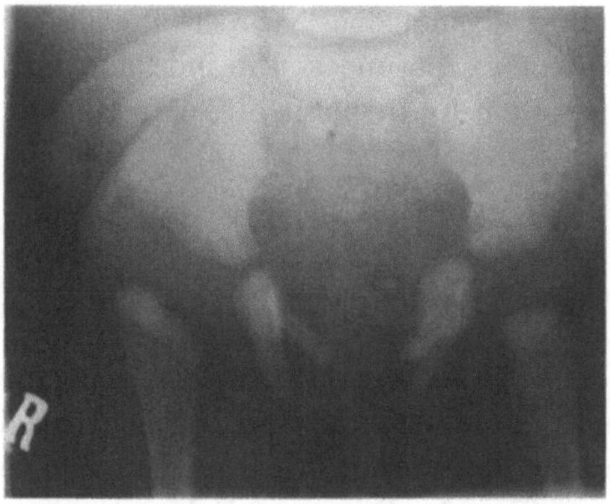

Fig. 1. Premature infant with dislocation of the right hip and multiple malformations and cystic kidney

* Department of Radiology at the Children's Hospital of the University of Erlangen-Nuremberg, Federal Republic of Germany

well as a significantly greater incidence in breech presentations and a tendency to higher involvement of the left side.

In the literature it is generally alleged that about 90% of all cases of dysplasia of the hip are diagnosed by Ortolani's sign, but we estimate this figure to be at most between 70% and 80%.

Only in cases where dysplasia of the hip occurs together with instability of the ligaments does a "click" or Ortoloni's phenomenon appear at birth or shortly thereafter (Freislederer). In about 75% of the cases where infants show this symptom, dysplasia of the hip will appear in X-rays after the third month of life. Fortunately, if left untreated dyplasia of the hip does not invariably lead to subluxation or dislocation of the hip, because of the strong propensity for spontaneous self-correction during infancy. However, healing is often imperfect and in later life the acetabulum becomes markedly slanted, leaving the femoral head only partially covered. This constitutes the main cause of premature arthrosis of the hip which is so frequently observed.

Since all other clinical symptoms, both positive and negative, such as external rotation of a lower limb, limitation of abduction, and above all, differences in the creases at knees and buttocks, yield only uncertain hints for early diagnosis of dysplasia of the hip and moreover since the negative effects of Ortolani's phenomenon on the cartilagineous acetabulum are controversial, it is important to establish or to verify the diagnosis by radiologic examination.

In the literature, a great many radiologic criteria have been proposed for early diagnosis and detection of dysplasia of the acetabulum. Several authors have even proposed routine radiologic screening examination for early recognition of the disorder. The German Radiologic Society, however, has declined endorsement of any universal radiologic examination for all newborn infants because of the concomitant increment in genetic radiation exposure.

From the standpoint of pediatric radiology, our primary responsibility in a problematic situation is to describe the most advantageous X-rays techniques, to warn against increased unnecessary radiation exposure, and to indicate which radiologic findings we consider to be important for dysplasia of the acetabulum in early infancy, as well as to point out possilities of error.

X-Ray Technique

The infant is immobilized in a Babix device, the most dependable type being the flexible shell with a flat back that rests securely on the X-ray table. Special attachments make it possible to fasten the legs in the correct position and to correct lordosis by an abdominal strap (Fig. 2). When no Babix device is available, one or two assistants are needed to immobilize a restless infant (Fig. 3).

The X-ray is taken in the supine position with the lower limbs extended, the patellae pointing upward and the distal end of the feet rotated slightly internally to correct the anteversion of the femural neck. The central ray is directed onto

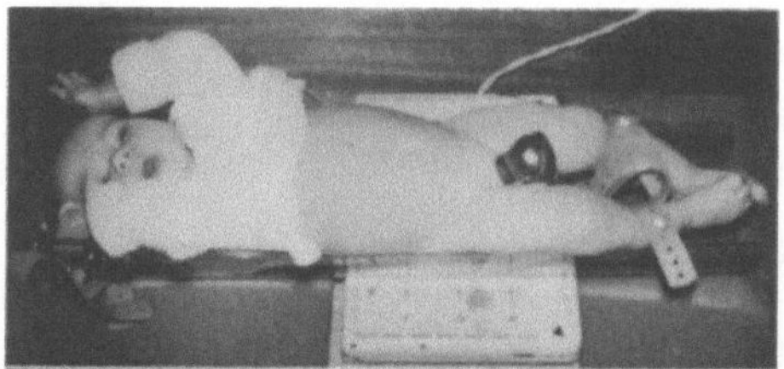

Fig. 2

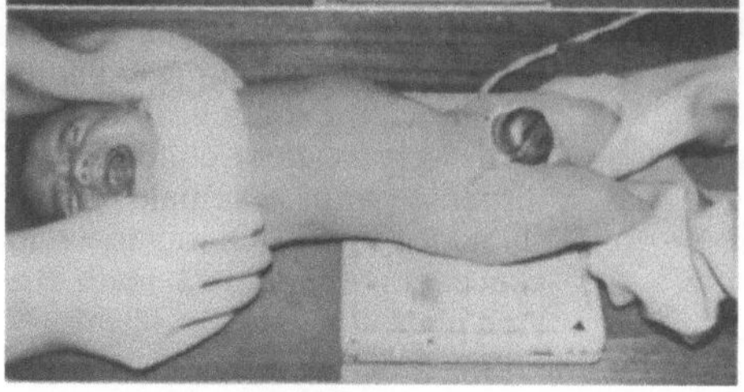

Fig. 3

Fig.2. Infant immobilized in a Babix device with flat support. The film cassette is contained in the Iontomat cassette. No secondary radiation diaphragm

Fig. 3. Infant immobilized by two assistants holding the lower limbs extended, the patellae pointing upward, the toes rotated slightly internally

the median line of the body slightly above the symphysis pubis, with the film-focus distance generally set at 1–1.15 m.

In order to keep the radiation dosage at the lowest possible level, the following precautions are recommended:

1. The use of heavily reinforced (special) casettes, which reduces radiation exposure by 50% in comparison with standard shields.
2. Omission of the Bucky diaphragm, which would intensify the radiation dosage by 15%–20%. Since the bone structure has no significance for evaluation of dysplasia of the acetabulum, a secondary radiation diaphragm can be dispensed with. The infant is placed instead with the buttocks directly over the X-ray casette, on using automatic exposure on film contained within the so-called Iontomat casette.
3. Secure adjustment of the gonad shield is a must. For male infants, a tightly fitting lead capsule serves to protect the gonads, although protection depends on whether the testes have descended or not. While still in the inguinal canal, the testes cannot be protected, but when they have already descended into the scrotum, protection can be practically total. In cases where the testes have not yet descended, an effort can be made to draw them into the scrotum before an X-ray is taken, a rubber band is placed around the scrotal neck to keep the testes from reascending into the inguinal canal as a result of a cremasteric reflex (Fendel).

For females, a properly positioned lead shield can also lessen the radiation dosage for female gonads by 70%–80%. One must allow for the fact, however, that the ovaries are placed relatively high in newborns and very young infants, usually within the greater pelvic area or even higher. The lead shield must therefore extend sufficiently high, with the umbilical area serving as a guideline. The

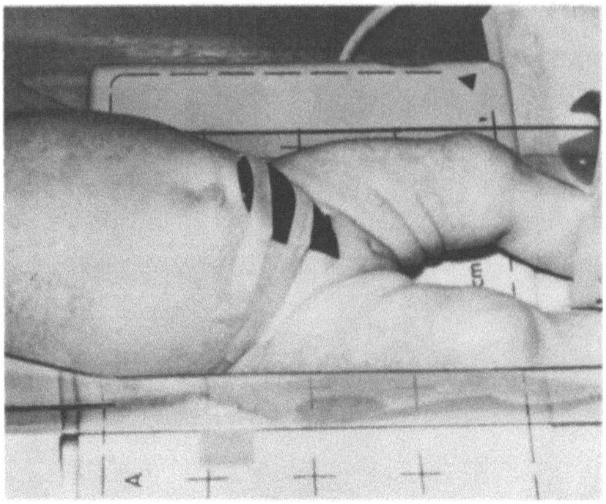

Fig. 4. Application of a female gonad shield, extending cranially as far as the umbilical region. With very restless children, we dispense with a female gonad shield for the first X-ray to avoid concealing one hip beneath the lead plate

most adaptable shields are 1-mm-thick triangular lead patches cut to order in various sizes as needed and secured in place with adhesive tape (Fig. 4). For examination of newborns, which we do not recommend because of the uncertain evidence obtained, the X-ray technique used by Andren and von Rosen is suggested. The children are immobilized in the supine position, with both lower limbs abducted to 45° and rotated slightly internally, so that on the picture obtained the longitudinal axis drawn through the upper thigh does not fall lateral to or above the lateral portion of the roof of the acetabulum.

Radiation Exposure from Pelvic X-Rays During Infancy

For several years it has been possible in nearly all radiologic examinations to ascertain the amount of radiation exposure, both in each individual case and in the total casework among all patients, by the simple method of recording patient exposure in the form of surface dosage incidence, using the measure $r \times cm^2$. The product of $r \times cm^2$ will always remain constant, even when the focus and the object are at varying distances, because the density of radiation decreases by the square of the distance, whereas the area of the concomitant radiation pyramid increases. When evaluating this parameter, though, one must bear in mind that measurement of surface dosage incidence does not constitute a true measurement in the strict sense of dosimetry. It is not a measurement of the dosage absorbed by the body but solely for the level of energy, that is, the quantity of radiation emitted by an X-ray tube with a field of fixed size in an individual examination.

In evaluating the surface dosage in 159 pelvic X-rays during infancy (Schellmann and Schuster), we obtained the following values: about $5 \ r \times cm^2$ from the third to the sixth month of life and about $7 \ r \times cm^2$ from the seventh to the twelfth month, values that agree by and large with those arrived at by Fendel.

By measuring the gonadal dosage, while observing the above-mentioned radiation protection precautions, we arrived at the following estimates: a gonadal dosage of 0.3–0.5 mrad for a single pelvic X-ray of a male, measured directly next to the gonads, and considerably less with a secure lead capsule; for a female, with a somewhat insecure gonad shield, the estimates fluctuated from 1–5 mrad during the first year of life. If we assume normal radiation exposure to be about 100 mrad/year (that is, 0.3 mrad/day), the female gonadal dosage for a single pelvic X-ray corresponds to a normal radiation exposure of 8–10 days; without a gonad shield, to a normal radiation dosage of 20–30 days. In males, with a secure gonad shield, the gonadal dosage lies within a range of several hours on a scale of normal dosage (Table 1).

Table 1. Radiation exposure of the most important radiologic examinations during childhood (Fendel) compared with normal radiation exposure per annum. The amounts given correspond to the amounts of surface exposure found by us. The table shows that the gonadal dosage for a pelvic X-ray with a secure gonad shield is no greater than for a chest X-ray

% of surface dosis of normal radiation exposure per annum		Gonadal dosis as time period per normal radiation exposure per annum
Pelvic X-ray (infant without diaphragm)	< 1%	2–3 hours (males, with gonad shield) 20 days without gonad shield
Chest X-ray	< 1%	2–3 hours
Flat plate of the abdomen with diaphragm	5%	70 days with gonad shield
Skull in 2 planes with diaphragm	15%–20%	10–12 hours (males, with gonad shield)

Use of an indirect technique – that is, of a 70 or 100-mm camera lens to photograph the final picture taken from the image-intensifier – permits a saving in radiation dose of about 90%, in comparison to standard X-rays with the usual combination of film and plate. However, to date this technique is available only at special X-ray centers.

Radiologic Criteria for Evaluation of Dysplasia of the Hips

Our research has enabled us to confirm the prevalent assertions in the literature with respect to early radiologic diagnosis during the first 3 months of life. Only cases with striking clinical findings, such as subluxation or dislocation, can be distinguished radiologically. In such cases, one can visualize an elevation and lateralization of the femur on standard X-rays (see Fig. 1). Evaluation of dysplasia of the acetabulum among newborns and during early infancy presents substantial difficulties since ossification is still incomplete. Using standard X-ray techniques, we were able to verify radiologically only 65 cases of suspected "dysplasia of the hip" among 100 newborns and infants under 4 months of age who had Ortolani's sign or limited abduction. In this group we evaluated mainly the angle of the acetabular roof, which we took (following Schmidt) to be normally 26° ±5° in newborn males and 30° ±3° in females.

For newborns, the X-ray technique suggested by Andren and von Rosen, that is, with the lower limbs brought into 45° abduction, yielded better results, and 40 cases among 48 children with a "click" could be substantiated radiologically. In general, though, our findings demonstrate the undependableness of early radiologic diagnosis before the fourth month of life. Radiologic findings are scantier among newborns and during early infancy, apparently, than the findings from examination for Ortoloni's sign and tests for limitation of abduction. Only after the third month is ossification of the acetabulum sufficiently advanced to permit detection of retarded ossification or development and of a possible dysplasia of the acetabular roof.

After the third month of life, we try to diagnose dysplasia of the hip first by deviations in development of the acetabular roof. Therefore it is important to know what form the acetabulum assumes at each stage of life. The most crucial criteria to be remembered during evaluation of the development of the acetabulum in each successive age group are: *formation of the lateral rim of the*

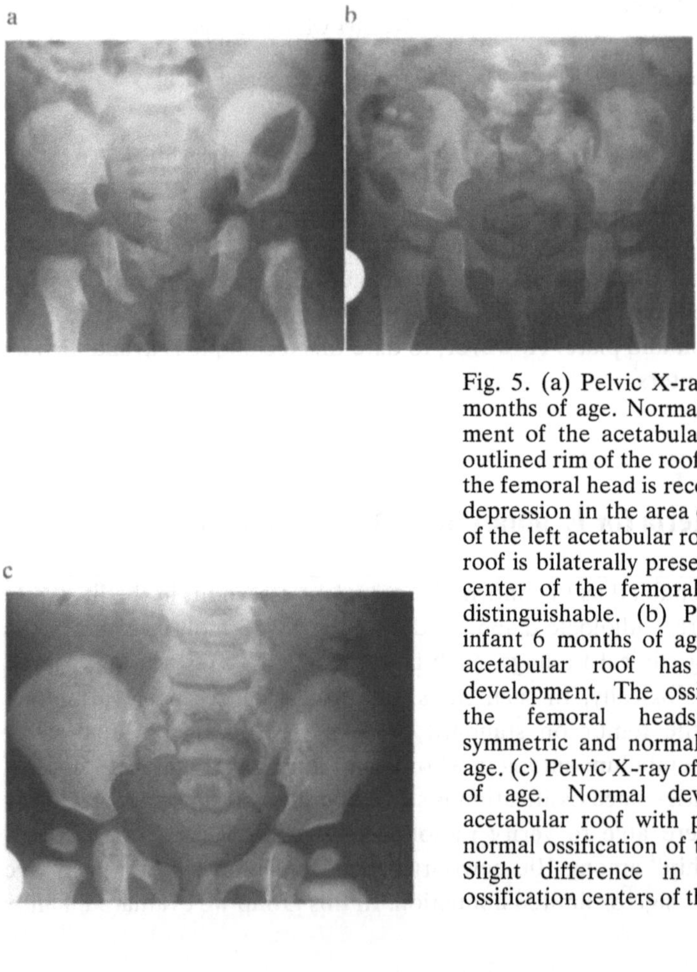

Fig. 5. (a) Pelvic X-ray of an infant $3^1/_2$ months of age. Normal bilateral development of the acetabular roof and sharply outlined rim of the roof. The impression of the femoral head is recognizable as a small depression in the area of the median third of the left acetabular roof. The vault of the roof is bilaterally present. The ossification center of the femoral heads are barely distinguishable. (b) Pelvic X-ray of an infant 6 months of age. The arch of the acetabular roof has normal bilateral development. The ossification centers of the femoral heads are bilaterally symmetric and normally located for that age. (c) Pelvic X-ray of an infant 9 months of age. Normal development of the acetabular roof with proper arching and normal ossification of the rim of the roof. Slight difference in size between the ossification centers of the femoral heads

acetabular roof, steepness of the angle of the acetabulum, vaulting of the acetabular roof, and the *impression of the femoral head* on the acetabular roof. Normal formation of the rim of the acetabular roof usually takes place during the third to fourth months, so that the acetabular roof is laterally defined by a relatively sharp border (Fig. 5 a).

In most cases of retarded development, a small round recess in the acetabular roof will appear in the area of transition to the lateral border of the ala ossis ilei, as shown in Figure 6. Children with such a hypoplasia of the rim of the acetabular roof without other roof symptoms carry a good prognosis for spontaneous healing.

At the beginning of the fourth month of life, the acetabular roof begins to form a vault, which becomes more pronounced in the fourth and fifth months, so that the border of the acetabulum develops a shallow arch. Methods of measurement to determine the arch of the acetabular roof are described by Marchese et al. (Figs. 5 a–c).

Even before the cartilagineous femoral head has become ossified, it can already be discerned as a tiny cavity or at least a depression in the area of the border of the acetabular roof. In pathologic cases, this depression occurs in the lateral third of the roof (Doberti and Manhood).

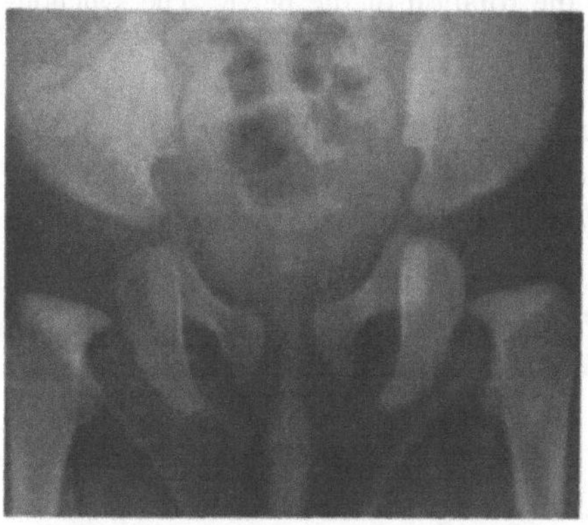

Fig. 6. Pelvic X-ray of an infant $3^1/_2$ months of age. The acetabula are relatively shallow on both sides. The rims of the acetabular roof are not yet sufficiently ossified. Small recesses can be seen at transition from the acetabulum to the lateral border of the corpus ossis ilei

The steepness of the acetabulum and the angle of its roof have always been cited as the most important parameters for detection of dysplasia. Tönnis' measurements of the angle of the acetabular roof in normal infants showed its constant decrease during the first year of life. We were unable to fully substan-

Table 2. Mean values and 2-sigma deviations of the angle of the acetabulum from the 1st to the 4th trimester of life. Evaluation of 253 normal pelvic X-rays in infancy

Age	Mean values	2-sigma deviation
1–3 months	24.4	7.3
4–6 months	23.1	6.3
7–9 months	21.9	7.4
10–12 months	20.2	9.0

tiate this constant decrease of the angle of the acetabular roof during infancy. Out of 253 pelvic X-rays of normally developed infants from birth to 1 year of age we calculated mean values and their 2-sigma deviations for the acetabular angle (Table 2). Accordingly, we consider a 30° angle to be normal during the first two trimesters of life and a 28° angle during the third trimester.

The very process of measuring the angle, though, contains the danger of misdiagnosis, because of many technical radiologic conditions which can affect the magnitude of the angle (Sinios, Ball). As often observed, a slight lateral rotation of the pelvis is sufficient to alter the angle of the acetabulum. On the side where the transverse diameter of the ilium is seen to be narrowed, the cartilagineous union between the ischium and pubis appears to be enlarged, as does the angle of the acetabular roof (Fig. 7).

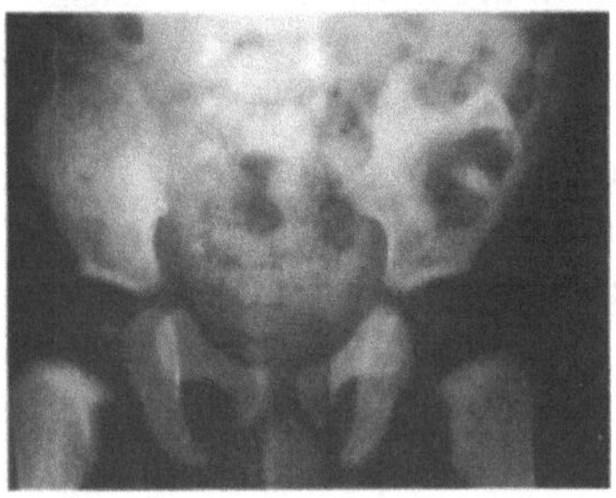

Fig. 7. Pelvic X-ray of an infant 5 months of age. A slight leftward rotation of the pelvis causes the left ala ossis ilium to appear wider than the right. On the side of the narrower ala ossis ilium the angle of the acetabulum appears slightly larger due to the rotation of the pelvis. The synchondrosis ischiopubica appears larger on this side

Even the pelvic slant observed in kyphosis and lordosis of the lumbar spine has a decided effect on the angle of the acetabular roof. As a measurement for determining the associated pelvic slant, we found the index proposed by Ball to be reliable: If we designate the longest vertical diameter of the obturator foramen as "a" and the distances between Hilgenreiner's line and the upper

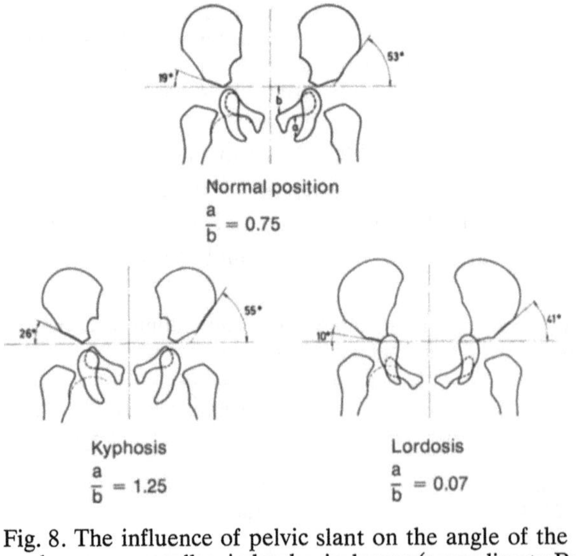

Fig. 8. The influence of pelvic slant on the angle of the acetabular roof. In lordosis the angle appears smaller, in kyphosis, larger (according to Ball)

margin of the superior ramus of the pubis as "b," then the quotient $^a/_b$ expresses the index. In a normally positioned pelvis, the index is 0.75/1.0. In practice this means that the segments should appear to be more or less of the same length on the X-ray. Lordosis leads to a reduction of the index, kyphosis to an increase. In pronounced cases of lordosis, the angle of the acetabular roof is noticeably smaller and in kyphosis it is larger, as shown by the schematic drawings of the pelvis in Figure 8, drawn from the original X-rays of a deceased infant whose pelvis had been slanted by varying degrees.

Only in doubtful cases do we use a goniometer to determine the exact angle of the hip joint. Otherwise, we employ evaluations by the above-named criteria, above all by the development of the acetabular roof at a given age. One should also bear in mind the well-known division of a dysplastic joint into wedge-shaped segments, as proposed by Schultheiss, which permits evaluation of the extent of anomalies in ossification (Fig. 9).

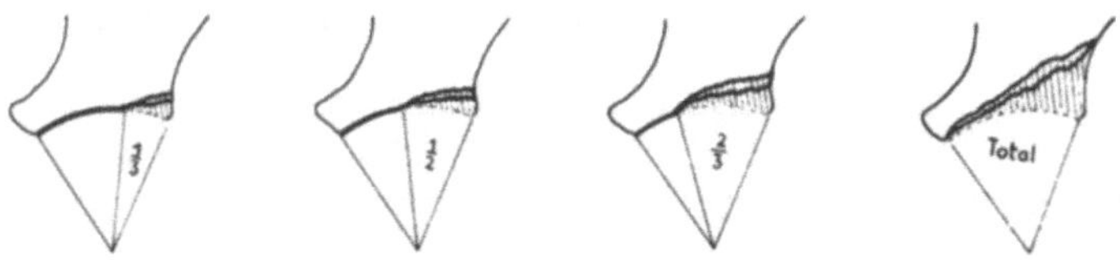

$^1/_3$ Wedge segment $^1/_2$ Wedge segment $^2/_3$ Wedge segment Total wedge segment

Fig. 9 Division of dysplastic acetabulum into wedge-shaped segments (according to Schultheiss)

Figure 10 (a–c) shows varying degrees of dysplasia of the acetabular roof in infants 4 months of age.

A delayed appearance of the ossification center of the femoral head or a difference in site of these centers are often overestimated as symptoms of

a b

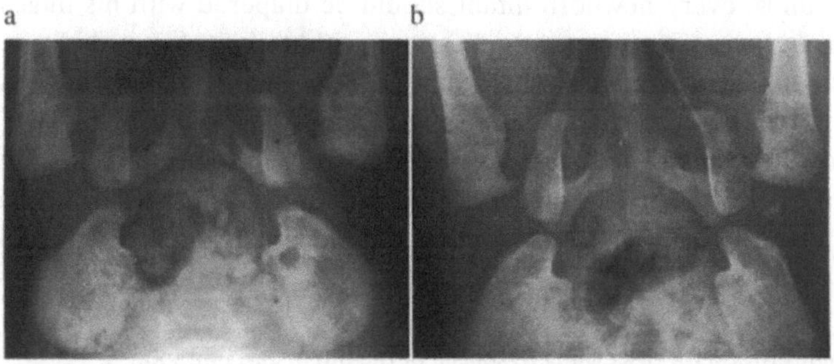

c

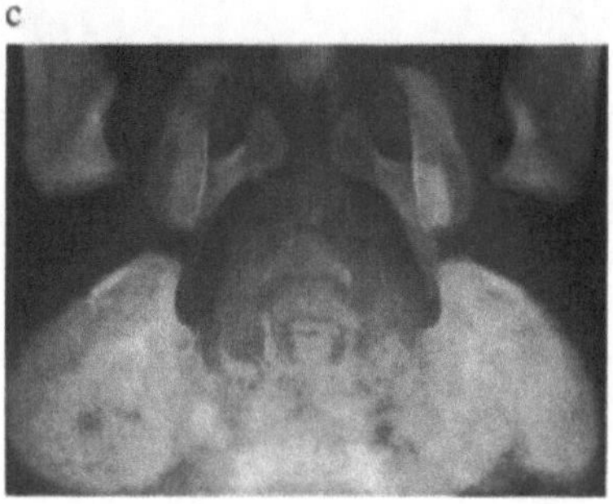

Fig. 10. (a) Pelvic X-ray of an infant 4 months of age. Slight lateral hypoplasia of the rim of the acetabular roof. (b) Pelvic X-ray of an infant 4 months of age. Dysplasia of the acetabulum with flattening of the cavity, increase in the angle of the acetabulum, and irregular ossification of the lateral portion of the acetabular roof. (c) Pelvic X-ray of an infant 4 months of age. Severe left-sided dysplasia with steeply angled acetabulum and incompletely developed acetabular roof. Slight right-sided dysplasia, also with increased angle of the acetabulum and hypoplasia of the rim of the acetabular roof

dysplasia of the hip. The formation of the bony nucleus of the femoral head can be delayed until the 10th month, even in a healthy child, and a slight difference in the size of the epiphyseal centers is often to be observed in perfectly normal hips. The sizes of the ossification centers of the femoral heads of normal infants have been ascertained by us as shown in Tables 3a and b.

Table 3a. Height of the ossification center of femoral heads during the first year of life (mean value and 2-sigma deviations)

Age	Mean value	2-sigma deviation
1–3 months	0.3	1.2
4–6 months	2.4	3.6
7–9 months	5.5	3.7
10–12 months	7.3	4.1

Table 3b. Width of the ossification center of femoral heads (mean value and 2-sigma deviations)

Age	Mean value	2-sigma deviation
1–3 months	0.4	1.9
4–6 months	3.8	5.7
7–9 months	8.3	5.1
10–12 months	10.9	5.9

In summary, we would like to recommend on the basis of clinical and radiologic examinations the following practical procedure in diagnosing dysplasia: On prophylactic grounds, every newborn infant should be diapered with his thighs widely apart since there are no certain indications, either clinical or radiologic, for the presence of dysplasia in earliest infancy. In cases with clinical symptoms during the first 3 months, abduction treatment should be undertaken.

We carry out radiologic examinations only after the third month of life. In evaluating them, the development of the acetabular roof in relationship to the given age is of greatest significance. The other radiologic criteria are shown in Table 4.

Table 4. Radiologic criteria for discerning dysplasia of the hip in early infancy

X-rays from the 4th month of life (only in exceptional cases earlier)
Acetabular roof angle (normal 27°–30°) Femoral head in medial, inferior quadrant Menard-Shenton's line (with reservations) CE-angle (normal up to at least 10°)

Table 5. Indications for radiologic examination of the pelvis to determine the presence of dysplasia of the hip in infancy

To be X-rayed:
1. All infants with clinical symptoms
2. All infants delivered by breech presentation
3. All infants with hereditary tendencies

For discussion: all infants in the 4th month of life by indirect technique (with 90% reduction in radiation)

We X-ray all infants with clinical indications, i.e., Ortoloni's phenomenon in newborns, limited abduction under 60°, hips that are too flaccid, external rotation of the lower limbs, differences in creases of the buttocks, lower limb shortening and any other symptoms of dislocation. In the fourth month of life, we also conduct radiologic examinations of all children who show no clinical symptoms but who were born by breech presentation or who may have hereditary tendencies (Table 5).

If it becomes possible on a larger scale to reduce the radiation exposure per X-ray, for example by the indirect technique mentioned above with 70 or 100-mm camera photographs of the image-intensifier picture, then the question of routine X-ray screening examinations as a precautionary measure should again be investigated. In this connection, data obtained by Freislederer from infants between 3 and 12 months of age are of interest. These infants presumably had no clinical indications of dysplasia or dislocation and were routinely X-rayed by means of an image-intensifier photograph. Among 1000 out-patient infants, 8 had subluxations or dislocations of the hip and 29 had dysplasia or retarded development of the acetabular roof. Among 1000 inpatient infants, 3 had subluxations or dislocations and 35 had dysplasia and irregular ossification of the acetabular roof.

Only by confident cooperation between pediatricians and orthopaedic surgeons can early recognition and appropriate and early treatment of this common discorder become a reality.

References

Ball, F., Kommenda, K.: Ann. Radiol. **11,** 298 (1968)
Doberti, A., Manhood, J.: Ann. Radiol. **11,** 276 (1968)
Ebel, K.-D., Willich, F.: Die Röntgenuntersuchung im Kindesalter. Berlin-Heidelberg-New York: Springer-Verlag 1968
Fendel, H., Goebel, W.: Ann. Radiol. **11,** 282 (1968)
Freislederer, W.: Röntgenologische Untersuchungen der Hüftdysplasie mit Hilfe der Bildverstärkerphotographie. Wiss. Kolloquium, Univ. Kinderklinik München, März 1973
Freislederer, W.: Personal communication
Marchese, G. S., Albini, G., Balocco, A., Grassi, E.: Ann. Radiol. **11,** 267 (1968)

Schellmann, B.: Patienten-Dosimetrie bei Röntgenuntersuchungen im Kindesalter. Inaugural-Dissertation Erlangen, 1970
Schmid, F.: Pädiatrische Radiologie, Bd. I. Berlin-Heidelberg-New York: Springer-Verlag 1973
Schultheiss, H.: Z. Orthop., Beiheft 100 (1965)
Sinios, A.: Pädiat. Prax. **8**, 641 (1969)
Vogt, S.: Röntgenanatomische Beckenmaße im Säuglingsalter. Inaugural-Dissertation Erlangen, 1969

English translation from the German edition *Der Orthopäde,* Vol. 2, pp. 219–225 (1973),

Femoral Osteotomies For Congenital Hip Dislocation

H. Wagner*

It is almost obligatory that congenital dislocation of the hip be accompanied by femoral neck axis deviation, i.e., by pathologic valgus and exaggerated anteversion. This axis defect should be corrected, whether the cause be a severely deficient acetabular roof over the femoral head, an increasing growth eccentricity of the capital epiphysis, or a lateralization or luxation tendency of the femoral head. Correction of the antetorsion then becomes more important than that of the valgus.

A. The Intertrochanteric Osteotomy

Because of technical difficulties of osteosynthesis, in many surgical centers, the femoral neck defect is being resolved simply by subtrochanteric osteotomy. For its stabilization, special thin medullary nails are driven from the tip of the greater trochanter, through the trochanter and its epiphyseal line into the medullary canal. This antiquated method is to be rejected, even though it is still in wide use and is still being described in the more recent literature.

The correction of the femoral neck defect should only be done at the intertrochanteric level, because the lesser trochanter, when in correct position, becomes pathologically retroverted through a subtrochanteric osteotomy. Also, through the broader surfaces of the higher osteotomy (intertrochanteric versus subtrochanteric), the distal fragment can be displaced medially and can therefore be more securely held with better means of fixation.

In children, when performing osteosynthesis at the proximal end of the femur, it is absolutely essential to avoid the epiphyseal line of the greater trochanter which can create growth deviation of the femoral neck, and especially of the capital epiphysis (Fig. 1). This applies equally to medullary nails, which are drilled from the tip of the trochanter through its growth line, and to right-angled blade-plates, which enter from the lateral aspect, crossing the growth

* Orthopädische Klinik des Wichernhauses (Surgeon in Chief: Prof. Dr. H. Wagner) Nuremberg/Altdorf, Federal Republic of Germany

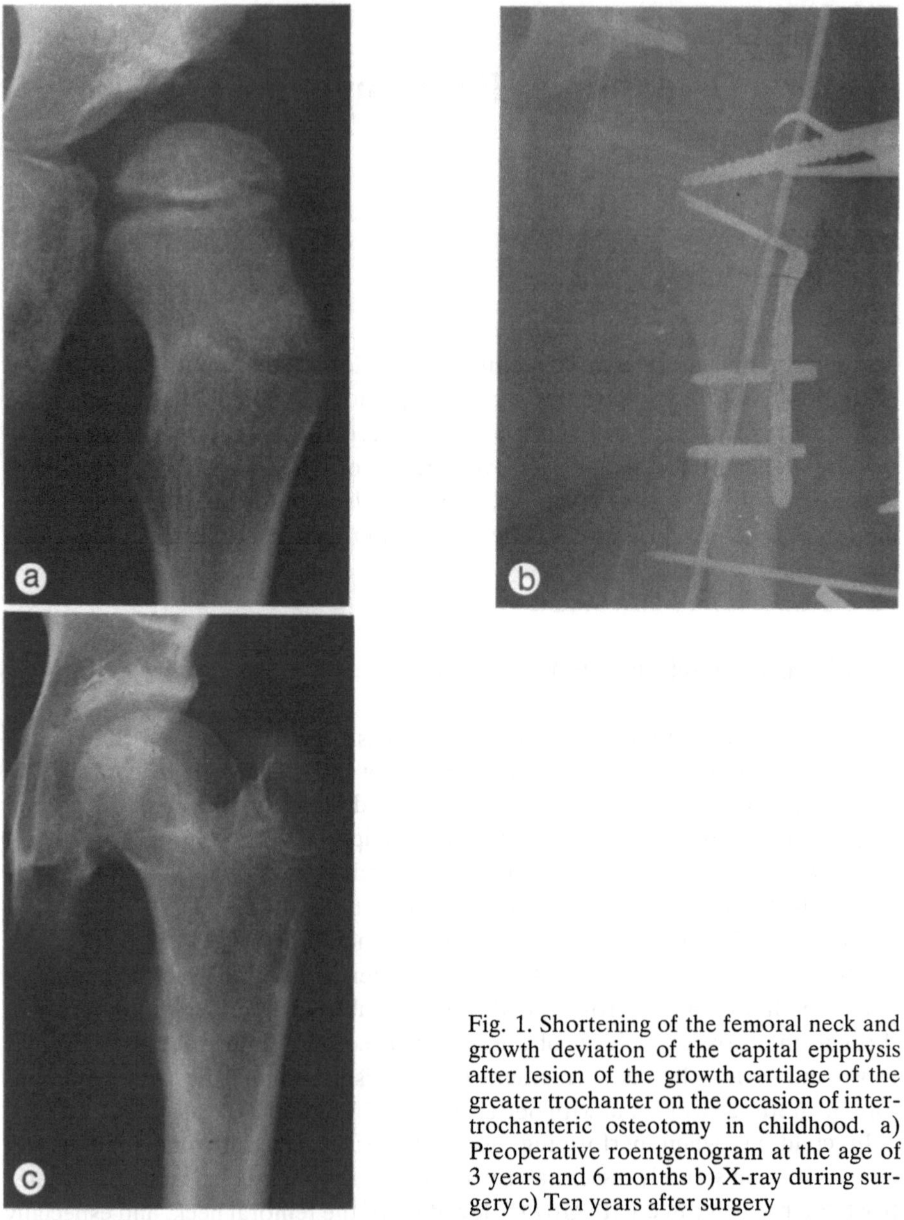

Fig. 1. Shortening of the femoral neck and growth deviation of the capital epiphysis after lesion of the growth cartilage of the greater trochanter on the occasion of intertrochanteric osteotomy in childhood. a) Preoperative roentgenogram at the age of 3 years and 6 months b) X-ray during surgery c) Ten years after surgery

cartilage. It should be mentioned that in osteosynthesis done in childhood, the growth line of the femoral neck should be avoided as well as the hip joint space itself. The effects of injury to the cartilaginous structures in children's hips only show up later, both clinically and radiologically, but they have an ominous functional and prognostic meaning and must not be minimized.

The exact planning and measuring of the proper size of the implant to be used and of the method chosen for the osteosynthesis of the proximal end of the femur must be carefully studied preoperatively. The stability of the osteosynthesis should be assured in order to attain maintenance of the correction; at the same time the implants used to assure this stability should be inserted with the least trauma so as to avoid as much damage as possible to the living bone. It must be further stressed that, in childhood, bone spongiosa is particularly delicate and after a previous operative procedure, appreciable bone atrophy can ensue.

For the intertrochanteric osteotomy the lateral approach is used. The skin incision descends the lateral aspect of the hip from the greater trochanter distally to the upper thigh. The fascia lata is split lengthwise, in the direction of its fibers, and the borders retracted with self-retaining retractors. The vastus lateralis, now exposed, is mobilized forward from behind, lifting it from the tendon of the gluteus maximus and the lateral intermuscular septum, as well as the coadjacent linea aspera. The origin of the M.vastus lateralis is cut obliquely about 1 cm distal from the tuberculum innominatum, following which this muscle is further mobilized by lifting it anteriorly, exposing the underlying femur. The site of the osteotomy is determined and marked by a fine chisel-cut at the level of the upper edge of the lesser trochanter. At the site of the intended osteotomy, a circumferential subperiosteal exposure of the bone should be done in order to avoid soft-tissue injury and bleeding, while distally from here, the lateral aspect of the femur should be exposed as little as possible.

There is a simple, dependable method for proper orientation of the proximal end of the femur after intertrochanteric osteotomy: before performing the actual osteotomy, the proximal end of the femur is brought into the desired corrected position by abduction and internal rotation of the lower limb (in cases of atypical or additional defect, a variation of this position may be necessary) confirming this position by X-ray or intensive image control. A thin 3 mm Steinmann pin or Kirschner wire parallel to the operating room floor is then inserted, at right angles to the median line of the patient. This is passed through the lateral cortex of the femoral shaft (just distal to the greater trochanter and its growth line) medially along the axis of the femoral neck up to, but not penetrating, the epiphyseal line of the femoral head (see Fig. 4b).

Both planes of orientation (median body line of the patient and the plane of the floor) can be judged accurately during operation; once the intertrochanteric osteotomy is performed parallel and distal to the Kirschner wire, the corrected position of the femoral neck can be judged and reexamined with precision, before finalizing with the osteosynthesis.

Osteosynthesis in Childhood

In the literature a great number of methods of osteosynthesis of the intertrochanteric osteotomy in childhood are quoted, from simple encircling wires over crossed Kirschner fixation-wires to stabilization with angle-plates. While we recommend certain well-proven procedures, other methods showing insufficient stability or severe traumatization we cannot.

External fixation using Schanz screws represents the simplest method of osteosynthesis. This operative procedure is relatively much easier than an internal (i.e., open) osteosynthesis, and avoids the necessity of a second operation for implant removal, since the Schanz screws can be removed without anesthesia. For intertrochanteric derotations and varisations, a Schanz screw is inserted proximal, and another distal, to the osteotomy site, and as close as possible to the latter (to avoid tilting of the osteotomized fragments). Then the proximal screw is gradually tightened into position while the distal screw, inserted into a previously made drill-hole, is tightened in a direction parallel to the transverse axis of the knee joint. At this point, the direction of the two screws enclose the angle of correction of the proposed wedge osteotomy. The latter is now cut between the two screws, and in patients where the bone is hard an entire wedge, with its base medially, is removed. Where the bone is soft, a smaller-angled wedge should be removed and the coadjacent bone edges impaled or compressed on each other subsequently.

On femoral neck axis correction, the proximal fragment is varisized and derotated, while the distal fragment is shifted medially at a distance of half the shaft's width, until the two screws become parallel. With the rigid external fixation apparatus (Müller, M. E.) interfragmentary compression can be applied through a screw mechanism, thus stabilizing the osteotomy site and assuring maintenance of position as well as promoting bone consolidation (Fig. 2).

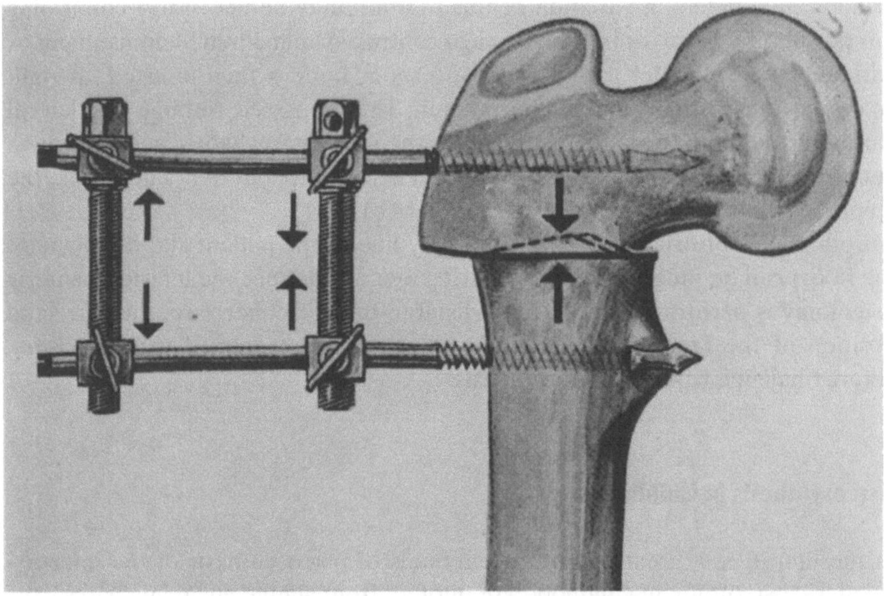

Fig. 2. External fixation for intertrochanteric osteotomy in childhood by the use of percutaneously applied Schanz screws. Interfragmentary compression is achieved with the Müller compression apparatus (from: Müller, M. E., Allgöwer, M. and Willenegger, H.: Manual of Internal Fixation, Springer, Berlin–Heidelberg–New York 1970)

Around each screw, the skin puncture wound must be sufficiently large and the intervening skin between the screw holes sufficiently loose, lest mechanical pressure or tension on the skin by the screws lead to skin necrosis with subsequent infection along the screw channels into the adjacent soft tissue. Each wound edge which will be in contact should be undercut on a slant away from the screw, and the small excess excised in order to assure sufficient looseness.

This osteosynthesis fixation via percutaneous Schanz screws alone is insufficient, necessitating additionally, a hip spica cast. The screws must not be incorporated; instead they should lie freely within the plaster. The femur can then move freely within the cast as a result of movement induced by breathing or local muscle contractions. Otherwise, once included in the plaster – or merely coming in contact with it during the course of even small movements – the screws are liable to loosen in the bone, causing pain.

When intertrochanteric osteotomy is performed in children, the Schanz screws are removed after 5 weeks, but the plaster is opened only after 8 weeks.

The *advantages* of the method of percutaneous Schanz screw fixation lie in the fact that the operation is a much less formidable procedure than other osteosynthesis methods, since the bone only requires the exposure necessary for the osteotomy itself. The Schanz screws are anchored via skin punctures close to the osteotomy site, thereby eliminating any further bone exposure such as is required in the application of a bone plate. Furthermore, a second operation for removal of metal is unnecessary, since the screws can be easily removed, without anesthesia, at the time of a change of dressing. A further advantage is seen occasionally in cases requiring subsequent correction of the neck angle, when this is done without additional surgery, by merely loosening the external fixation apparatus from the screws, changing the angle of the Schanz screws to the desired extent, then retightening the apparatus.

One *disadvantage* is the more prolonged immobilization, induced by the necessity of a hip spica, than would be required if fixation were obtained with an inserted implant. In cases with more severe bone atrophy such as is seen following operative hip repositioning, it is very difficult or even impossible to achieve adequate immobilization with the Schanz screws method. When there is insufficient area of contact between the osteotomized surfaces, the fragments may tilt, since the Schanz screws stabilize only in the frontal plane, offering insufficient resistance to tilting in the sagittal plane. Only when a wide area of contact exists can axial compression afford sufficient stability against tilting between the screws. A further disadvantage is that the screws maintain contact with the exterior relatively close to the operative site, facilitating infection, particularly if web necrosis secondary to mechanical pressure occurs in the screw channels of the skin or adjacent soft tissue. Finally, a funnel-shaped depression is often left after removal of the Schanz screws, which increases in size during growth and leaves a distressingly ugly scar.

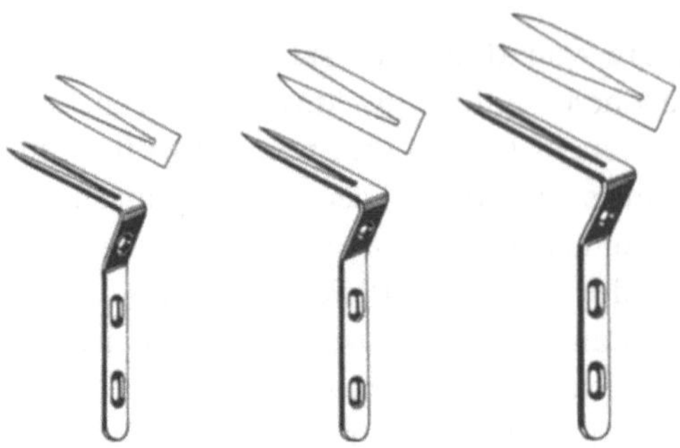

Fig. 3. The Altdorf hip clamp for intertrochanteric osteotomy in childhood. The clamp is available in 3 sizes. The proximal end of the blade is bifurcated and the blade itself is bent to make an angle of 130° with the plate

Osteosynthesis by Means of a Small Angle Plate in Childhood

It is our experience that, in children up to age twelve, osteosynthesis of an intertrochanteric osteotomy is most universally successful using an Altdorf hip clamp[1] (a modified Becker angle-plate) which, when screwed in situ, acts as a veritable clamp on the osteotomized fragments (Fig. 3). The proximal end of the blade is bifurcated and the blade itself is bent to make an angle of about 130° with the plate. The latter has two oval screw-holes in its shaft to allow leeway for blade shifting during compression, while distal to the angle is a round hole through which a screw is inserted into the proximal fragment. The metal of the plate is soft enough to permit changing the blade-plate angle when necessary, with a special bending instrument.

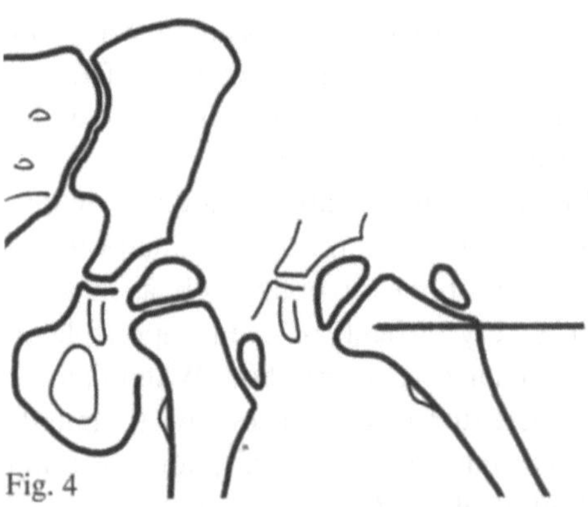

Fig. 4

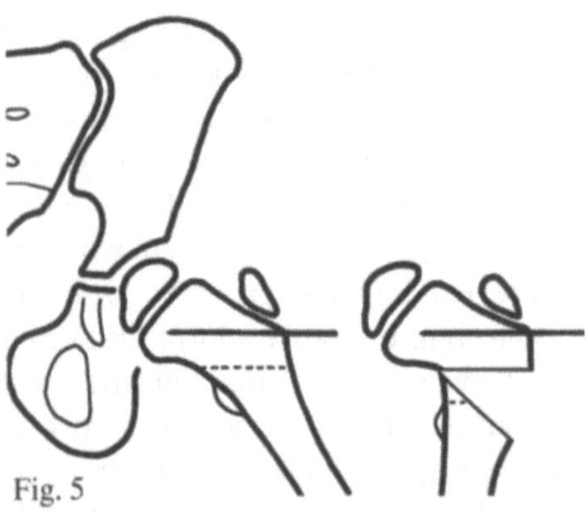

Fig. 5

Fig. 4. Intertrochanteric osteotomy. Before performing the actual osteotomy, the proximal end of the femur is brought into the desired corrected position just by abduction and internal rotation of the lower limb. A 3-mm-Steinmann pin is then inserted, parallel to the operating room floor and at right angles to the median line of the patient, just distal to the greater trochanter and its growth line

Fig. 5. The intertrochanteric osteotomy is executed in a superomedial direction, distal and parallel to the Steinmann pin. The correction is obtained by maintaining the Steinmann pin horizontal to the floor and at right angles to the median plane of the patient and bringing the distal fragment into neutral abduction-adduction and rotation. Through the open osteotomy cleft a medial bone wedge is removed from the distal fragment

[1] Manufactured by Aesculap, D-7200 Tuttlingen. Federal Republic of Germany.

The proximal femur is first oriented, placing the femoral neck in the corrected position with a 3-mm-thick Steinmann pin inserted distal to the epiphyseal line of the greater trochanter and directed along the femoral neck axis, all as previously described (Fig. 4). Then the intertrochanteric osteotomy is executed in a superomedial direction, distal and parallel to the Steinmann pin (Fig. 5). A slowly oscillating saw is very desirable since it is able to produce smoothly cut surfaces, thus permitting an accurate correction and stable contact of the osteotomized surfaces, especially important when dealing with atrophied bone.

Following osteotomy, the correction is obtained by maintaining the Steinmann pin horizontal to the floor at right angles to the median plane of the patient and bringing the distal fragment into neutral abduction-adduction (of the leg). The distal fragment at the osteotomy site is shifted medially about half of the shaft's width for two reasons:

1. Through the medial translocation, conditions for bone consolidation are improved. The proximal femur fragment with its asymmetrical configuration has a tendency to varus formation, or a bowing tendency at the osteotomy site. Through the medial transposition of the distal fragment, the proximal fragment becomes better supported medially and has its weight-bearing lever shortened. This diminishes the varus tendency and places the osteotomy surfaces under more direct pressure, which is necessary for bone healing.

2. The medial transposition diminishes a tendency for axis deviation of the distal fragment of the femur. Through derotation and varization of the femoral neck, the greater trochanteric mass is moved laterally, away from the median line which automatically leads to a varization of the limb axis. The medial transposition counteracts this.

Having adapted the osteotomy surfaces properly to each other, the osteosynthesis is started (Fig. 6). With careful hammer blows on a plate-holder instrument, the bifurcated blade of the angle-plate is forced proximally through the

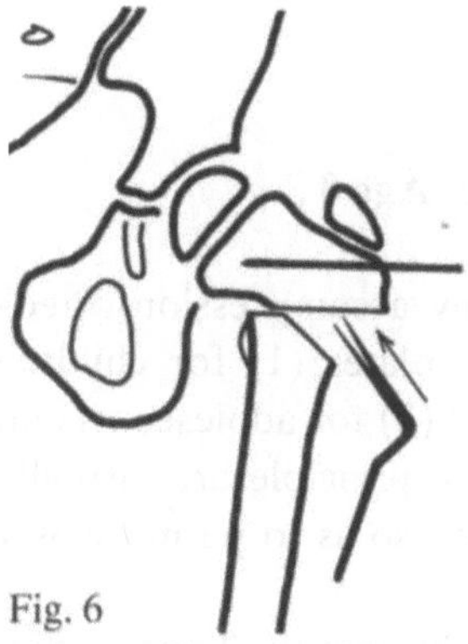

Fig. 6

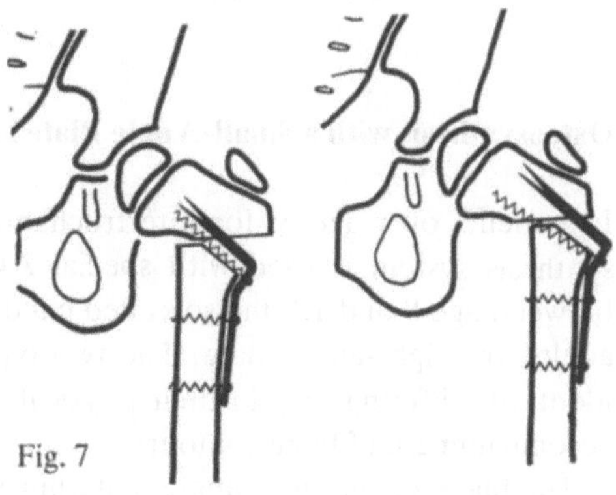

Fig. 7

Fig. 6. Internal fixation of intertrochanteric osteotomy. The bifurcated blade is forced into the cancellous bone osteotomy surface of the proximal fragment

Fig. 7. The further medial the blade of the angle-plate comes to lie in the proximal osteotomy surface, the stronger the medial translocation of the distal fragment becomes

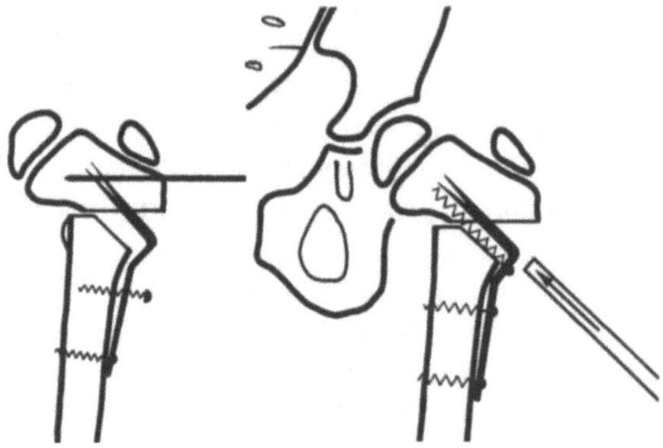

Fig. 8. Osteosynthesis for intertrochanteric osteotomy

spongy bone of the osteotomy surface into the proximal fragment until almost the entire blade is buried, i.e., almost to the angle of the plate. At this point, attention is called to the fact that the further medially the blade comes to lie in this osteotomy surface, the stronger the medial translocation of the distal fragment becomes (Fig. 7). Other methods of osteosynthesis using angle-plates have much less leeway for medial displacement.

After inserting the blade, leaving the proximal fragment in slightly less varus than required and the distal fragment slightly over-shifted medially, a slight overcorrection is made deliberately. This causes the distal tip of the plate to contact the femoral shaft, keeping the apex of the osteotomy cleft about 5–6 mm more distal than necessary (See Fig. 8). The interfragmentary compression is now gradually achieved, first by inserting and tightening a screw through the most distal hole in the plate and then successively in the more proximal hole, gradually pulling the distal fragment laterally to the plate, and bringing the proximal fragment into more varus. Now, after final inspection of the bifurcated blade, the most proximal lag screw is then gradually tightened into the proximal fragment, increasing even further the varus and the interfragmentary pressure (example in Fig. 9).

Osteosynthesis with a Small-Angle Plate in Patients over Age 8

In patients over age 8, for intertrochanteric osteotomy a compression osteosynthesis system is used with special AO right-angle plates (1) for children between age 8 and 12, the so-called child hip-plate and (2) for adolescents and adults, the right-angle plate. The two types of plates in principle are virtually identical, differing only in their physical profile and size so as to permit closer accompaniment of bone contours.

The blade of the right-angle plate must be inserted through the lateral corticalis into the proximal fragment. The bone channel for the blade is prepared or cut into the bone with a special seating chisel under X-ray control and is cut a little short of the final "driven-home" distance of the actual plate to allow for secure fit of the blade when it is finally impacted to its full length. Since the right-angle, as its name implies, shows a distinct angle of 90° between blade and plate, the intended correction angle of the osteotomy will be determined by "seating" this special chisel into the proximal fragment (Fig. 10). By angulating

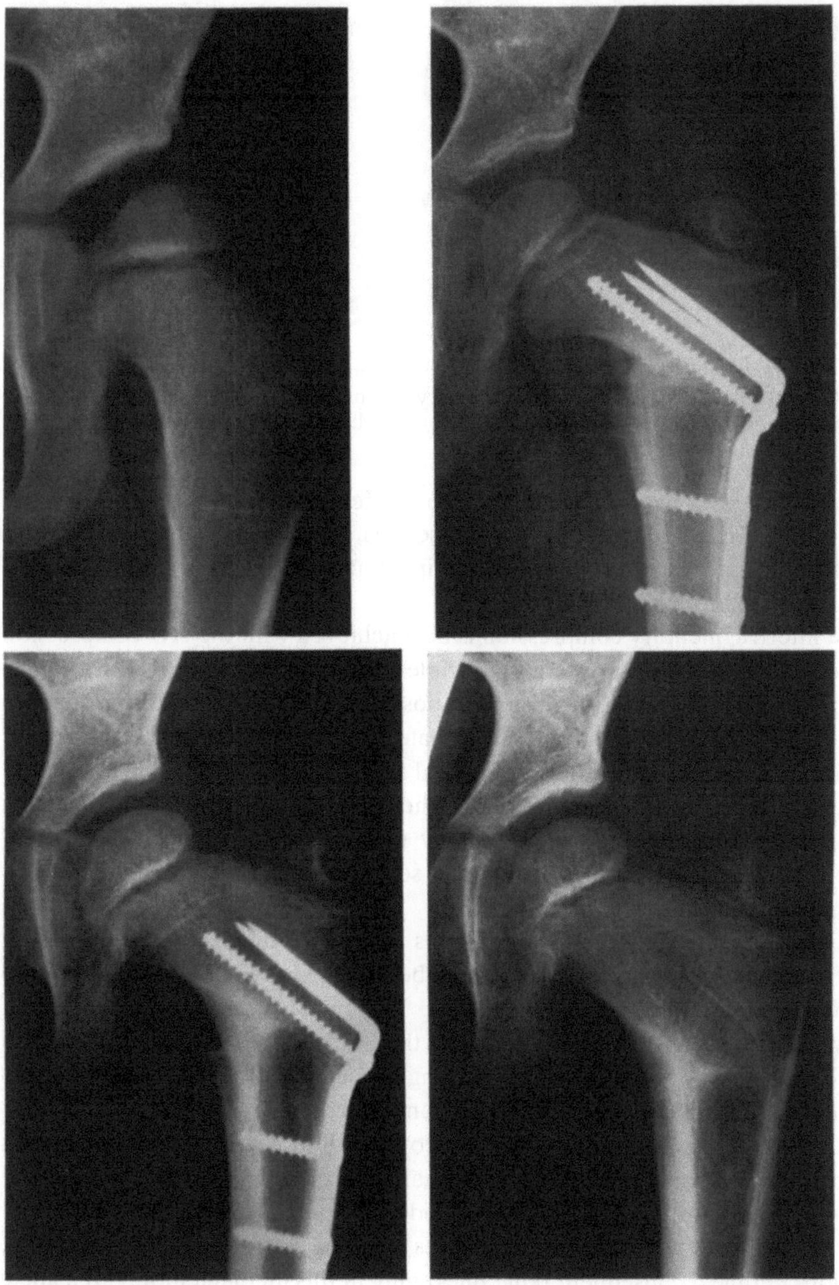

Fig. 9. Intertrochanteric osteotomy in a 4-year-old girl with acetabular dysplasia and exaggerated valgus and anteversion deviation of the femoral neck. X-rays 3, 6 and 18 months after surgery

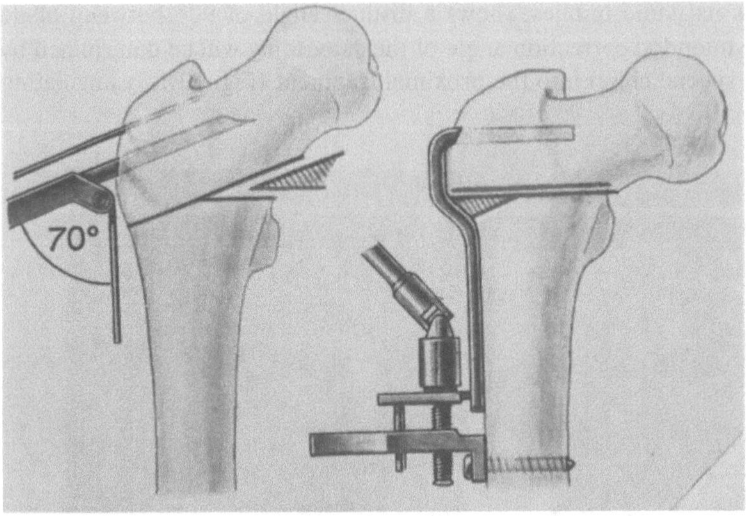

Fig. 10. Osteosynthesis for intertrochanteric osteotomy in adolescents and adults using the AO right-angle plate. The interfragmentary compression is achieved with the Müller compression device (from Müller, M. E., Allgöwer, M. and Willenegger, H.)

this chisel up or downward, in relation to the femoral long axis, and anteriorly or posteriorly in relation to the transverse axis, the proximal fragment will be shifted more into varus or valgus (as desired) and the distal fragments rotated internally or externally.

The interfragmentary compression is best achieved with the AO compression device, which works on the screw principle of a carpenter's jig. The jig is first loosened or unscrewed to its most open position. Then at one end, it is hooked into the last hole of the distal end of the plate, and through a hole at its other end it is firmly screwed to the adjacent femoral shaft. The jig is then slowly screwed to a closer position, and in doing so, via the blade plate, the femoral fragments are approximated, putting the osteotomy planes under pressure against each other. Then the distal fragment is firmly screwed to the plate. The jig is then loosened slightly and removed.

If only a short span of tightening suffices to produce the desired compression, a self-compressing (Allgöwer) plate may be used. A screw is first inserted into the narrow end of each oval screw-hole. The final turns of the cone-shaped screw-head force a shift of the plate to the screw head, so that the latter is forced into the widest diameter of the lengthwise oval screw-hole. This creates the desired self-compression at the osteotomy site.

In osteosynthesis more difficulty is encountered in correcting a more severe varus defect not only because of the unusual abnormal bone quality, but also due to the necessity for excision of a bone wedge. In such a severe varus deformity with its abnormal weight-bearing stresses bending the proximal femur, there develops in time a consequent bone thickening in this medial femoral area and a porosity in the contralateral corticalis. For a valgization osteotomy, the seating chisel should be inserted relatively more cranially in this soft spongiosa of the

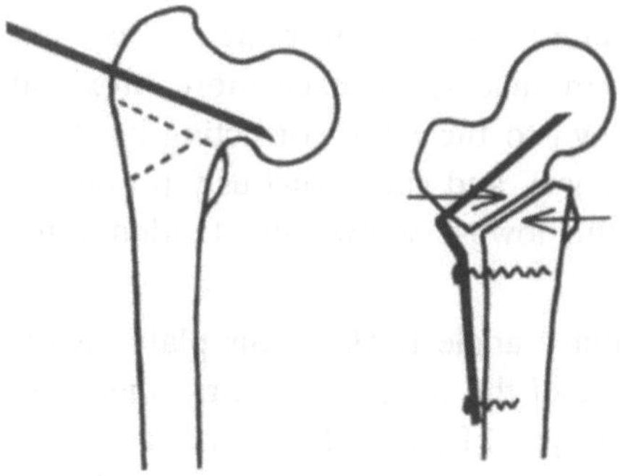

Fig. 11. Osteosynthesis for intertrochanteric valgization osteotomy using the 120° angle plate. The fragments are adapted with a slight overcorrection. By first inserting the most distal screw, and then, in succession – each more proximal screw, the distal fragment is gradually drawn to the plate producing interfragmentary compression

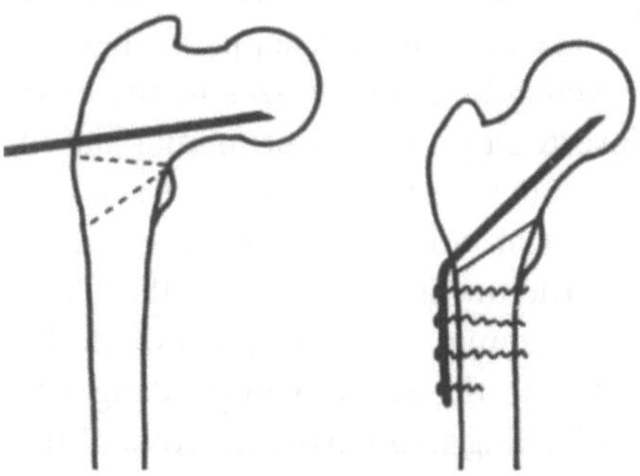

Fig. 12. Osteosynthesis for intertrochanteric valgization osteotomy using the 130° angle plate. Interfragmentary compression is achieved by the tension of the soft tissues. A medial buttress support of the fragments is absolutely necessary in order to avoid recycling bending stresses to the implant

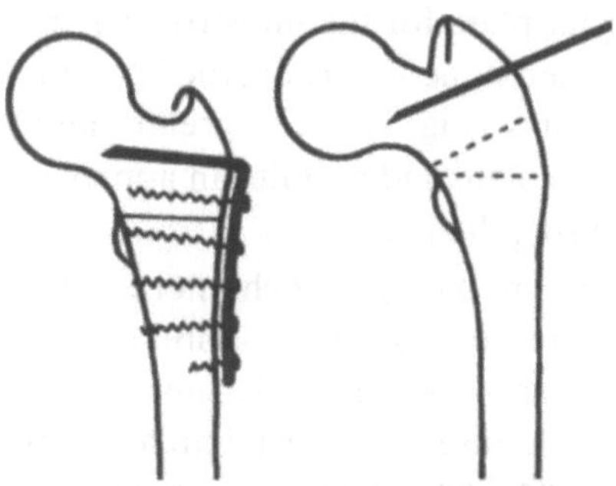

Fig. 13. Osteosynthesis for intertrochanteric valgization osteotomy using the condylar plate. The advantage of the condylar plate, especially in atrophic bone, is that firstly the anchoring of the plate to the proximal fragment is more secure, since the plate permits the insertion of one or two more screws cranial to the osteotomy, and secondly interfragmentary compression can be achieved with the jig-compression device

greater trochanter mass. With a right-angle plate, a strong tension stress should then occur at the outer aspect of the proximal fragment, which the atrophied bone therein cannot tolerate. It is then more appropriate to use the 120° angle-plate (Fig. 11) or in special cases, the 130° (Fig. 12) and in the most extreme cases the condylar plate (Fig. 13).

When using the 120° angle plate, the blade seating instrument should form an angle with the femur shaft which consists of the sum total of the desired correction angle plus the complementary angle of the plate of 60°. For a valgization of 30°, for instance, the seating chisel should be inserted at an angle of 90° to the femoral shaft. The intertrochanteric osteotomy ascending to medial, with the wedge based laterally, is then performed. Following this, the seating chisel is exchanged for the 120° angle plate. The fragments are adapted to each other with a slight overcorrection, that is, the distal fragment is slightly overshifted medially and the proximal fragment is slightly overvalgized. By first inserting the most distal screw and then, in succession, each more proximal screw, the distal fragment is gradually drawn to the plate correcting its slight overshift medially as well as the excess valgus, and simultaneously producing interfragmentary compression. Through the lowest screw, any tendency for plate shift cranially is prevented.

In the 130° angle plate the complementary angle is 50°. This plate also is inserted as previously described, but because of the steep blade angle there can be no appreciable compression action. This type of plate serves only as a support, in which case the interfragmentary compression must be established through soft-tissue tension. Therefore it becomes necessary to have dependable contact of the fragments on the medial side (medial buttress support), heightening the stability and thereby avoiding recycling bending stresses to the plate (Fig. 12). The blade of the plate must be inserted into the lower medial half of the femoral neck and head. Then the tip of the blade should come to lie immediately under the intersection of the compression and tension trajectories of the femoral neck. This is where the bone structure is thickest and the blade finds its best support. If the blade-tip is placed cranial to the intersection of the trajectories, the stability is much diminished, with the accompanying danger of injury to the locally arborizing blood vessels leading to a partial necrosis of the femoral head.

The most important advantage of the condylar plate for the intertrochanteric valgization osteotomy is that in a case of atrophied bone it permits the insertion of one or two more screws cranial to the osteotomy (Fig. 13). This creates more secure anchoring of the proximal fragment to the plate and permits an appreciable increase in interfragmentary compression, using the jig.

Particularly difficult problems are encountered in the intertrochanteric valgization osteotomy when the growth line of the greater trochanter is still open in children and adolescents particularly in coxa vara congenita. Because of the physical difference in size it becomes impossible to insert the thick implants into such small bones avoiding damage to the growth-line cartilage. In such cases Kirschner wires are useful. About 5–10 mm distal to the trochanteric epiphyseal line, three heavy Kirschner wires of 2.5 mm diameter are inserted into the femoral neck, parallel to its axis, reaching up to or close to the epiphyseal line of the caput. The intertrochanteric osteotomy is now performed, first without removal of a wedge (Fig. 14). In coxa vara congenita, at the level of the osteotomy on the medial or deep aspect of the femur one encounters exceptionally heavy fibrous connective tissue structure, which feasibly could render valgization of the femoral neck impossible. Therefore the osteotomy cut must be gradually pried open with a spreader and the medially situated heavy fibrous strings slowly spread apart or excised. This progressive resection is done with care so as to avoid the blood vessels normally traversing this area. As the thick fibrous tissue is gradually removed, the osteotomy cleft is more easily spread wider and wider, improving visualization and facilitating judgement of the soft tissue to be excised.

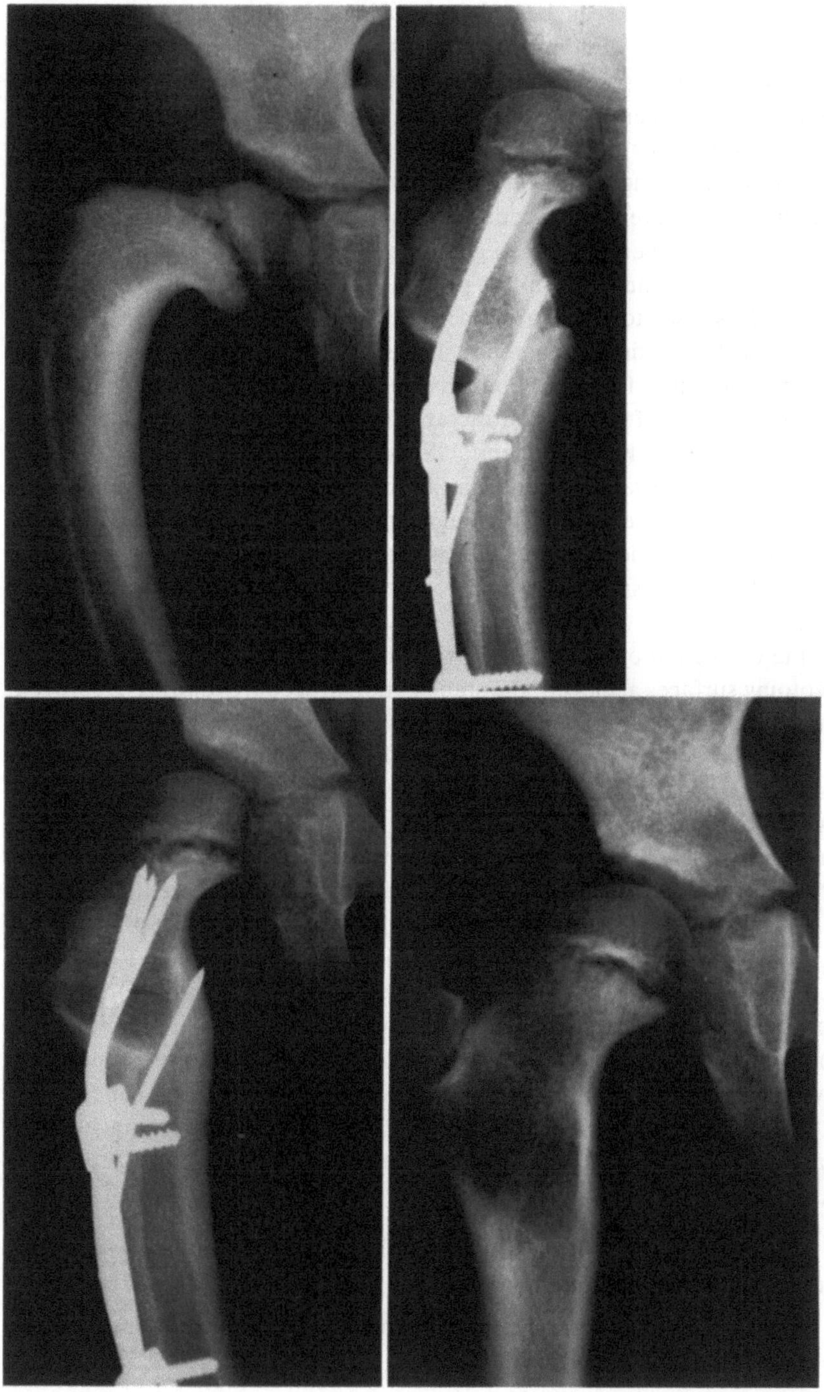

Fig. 14. Intertrochanteric valgization osteotomy for coxa vara congenita. Internal fixation with 3 heavy Kirschner wires. Radiographs of a 5-year-old girl at 3 months, 12 months and 3 years after surgery

Now the femoral neck can be valgized, using the Kirschner wires already inserted as a handle. It is of no purpose to try to help the correction of the femoral neck by leg abduction for this tightens the adductors, impeding any possible correction in this manner. Occasionally, it may even be necessary to perform an adductor tenotomy after closure of the wound.

The desired valgus angle is achieved by multiple small-wedge resections with an oscillating saw and repeated readaptations of the osteotomy surfaces, during which care must be taken to retain a good medial buttress. A simple, single, laterally-based wedge removed from the proximal or distal fragment, or even from both, is rarely satisfactory for a good correction. In most cases, a generous medial shift of the proximal fragment is necessary to the extent that the lateral cortex of the proximal fragment contacts the medial cortex of the distal fragment. When heavy, soft-tissue contractures are encountered, as in congenital deformity and especially in congenital femoral hypoplasia, a resection of a segment out of the distal fragment may be necessary to avoid too much soft-tissue resistance before adequate valgization is achieved. This resection-shortening for soft-tissue tension relief is also done in small stages, waiting a short time after each small resection to see when the tension has eased up sufficiently.

Once the correction of the femoral axis is obtained and proper adaptation of the osteotomy surfaces achieved, the stabilization procedure follows. To prevent subsequent shifting of the fragments, a Kirschner wire (1.5 mm diameter) is drilled in from the distal fragment, crossing the osteotomy cleft as far medially as possible. Its protruding end is bent down with pliers later to be attached lengthwise along the femoral shaft. The three previously inserted heavy Kirschner wires are also now bent downward individually until they maintain close contact with the outer aspect of the femoral shaft. These wires are then covered with a plate (semitubular plate), transversely curved on its deep surface to accompany the convexity of the femoral shaft, and secured thereto by short screws. Finally the vastus lateralis is reattached to its origin and sutured to the insertion of the gluteus medius via a strong weblike suture-line (tension-band suture). Such a strong reconstruction is particularly important to resist tension in the new valgus position. Thus an additional plaster spica is rendered superfluous.

The intertrochanteric osteotomy has advantages and disadvantages since there are four important biomechanical components being corrected simultaneously.

1. The correction of the femoral neck axis changes (direction and length) the lever arm of the pelvifemoral musculature.
2. The height of the greater trochanter controls the direction and tension of the pelvitrochanteric musculature.
3. The femoral neck axis influences the orientation of the femoral head and thereby its congruity with the acetabulum.
4. Change of direction of the femoral neck changes the local lines of stress, forcing a remodelling of the bone structure.

Intertrochanteric osteotomy can produce ideal conditions only where all four components show pathologic biomechanical values, and require correction in the same degree and direction. This, unfortunately, is not frequently the case. For instance, depending on the anatomic findings, the intertrochanteric osteotomy can improve the congruity of the joint surfaces and simultaneously bring about an aggravation in the pathologic height of the greater trochanter (Fig. 15). On the other hand, in a case of coxa valga with good congruity, the osteotomy will correct the former and worsen the latter (Fig. 16). For these reasons we must often compromise between the surgical indication and its method of cure.

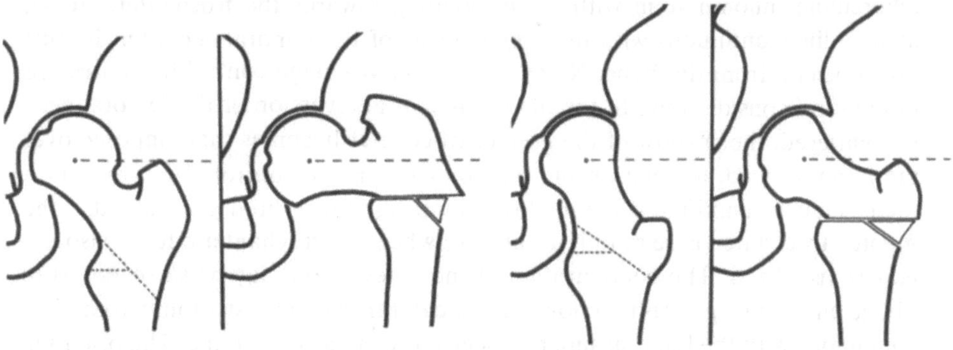

Fig. 15. Intertrochanteric varization osteotomy can improve the congruity of the joint surfaces and simultaneously impair the position of the greater trochanter

Fig. 16. In a case of coxa valga with good congruity, intertrochanteric varization can improve the orientation of the femoral neck and simultaneously worsen the congruity of the joint

On the other hand, intertrochanteric osteotomy is indicated in the correction of several associated defects of hip dislocation. Such a patient is often young, pain free, with no outwardly noticeable dysfunction as yet and the parents will probably require more than the usual amount of convincing regarding the surgical indication. We must then strive for a perfect mechanical restoration to justify the operative indication and to improve the prognosis of the hip joint as much as possible.

If the classic intertrochanteric osteotomy derotation varization cannot be expected to achieve perfect correction, then other methods of correction should tried.

B. Transplantation of the Greater Trochanter

Growth disturbances of the epiphysis of the femoral head and the epiphyseal line of the femoral neck in hip luxation Perthes' Disease, in post-traumatic and other disturbances can lead to a typical deformity, characterized by a severe femoral neck shortening and consequent affectation of the height of the trochanter. The joint surface of the femoral head in these cases often shows normal configuration and congruity. After an osteotomy of the greater trochanter with shifting to an anatomically more normal site, this deformity can be corrected.

The operation is performed via the lateral longitudinal approach. After splitting the fascia lata lengthwise, in the direction of its fibers, the vastus lateralis is detached from its origin at the tuberculum innominatum. The anterior border of the gluteus medius is exposed and a blunt elevator inserted on its deep surface pointing in the direction of the trochanteric fossa. For the proper orientation of the trochanter osteotomy, a Kirschner wire is inserted at the tuberculum innominatum with its tip pointing towards the trochanteric fossa, along a line continuous with the upper cortex of the femoral neck; but it must not protrude from the bone. X-ray with intensive-image control facilitates this orientation considerably. In the many cases of anteversion of the femoral neck encountered, the shadow of the greater trochanter becomes superimposed over the femoral head, as seen on the screen of the image control. The procedure, then, is much simplified when the lower limb is so far rotated internally that the greater trochanter is seen only in profile, when the trochanteric fossa also becomes visualized. The configuration of the anteversion may be so severe as to oblige one to change the direction of the greater trochanter osteotomy from a line continuous with the femoral superior neck cortex to a steeper line. The orienting Kirschner wire is brought into the corresponding direction with its tip almost in the trochanteric fossa, thus avoiding vessel injury and a possible necrosis of the femoral head.

A flat, blunt Hohmann retractor is applied to the back edge of the greater trochanter, pushing back and protecting the vascular dorsal tissues while the osteotomy is performed, preferably with an oscillating saw, following the distal side of the Krischner wires, stopping just short of the trochanteric fossa and thus avoiding reaching the vessels herein. A flat 3-cm-wide osteotome is now placed intracleft and its handle moved cranially, wedging open the osteotomy cleft and cracking through the corticalis in the cleft depths. With a slow contrary movement of the osteotome chisel, the osteotomy cleft is opened up medially and the greater trochanter slowly pushed away cranially. With a fine-toothed clamp, the greater trochanter is pulled even further laterally for more adequate visualization, permitting release of all adhesions between the subjacent joint capsule and the greater trochanter and its glutei. Often, because of the femoral neck foreshortening, the greater trochanter abuts close to the joint capsule, even when the X-ray has shown a space between femoral head and trochanter. Here the greater trochanter must be particularly carefully detached from the capsule (to avoid damage to the retinacular vessels). Sufficient mobilization of the trochanter will be recognized when the muscles respond elastically to pull. On the other hand, if pulling laterally and distally still elicits resistance, other adhesions should be looked for and detached.

The greater trochanter is now shifted laterally and distally, and in cases of accentuated anteversion, also ventrally. The new receptor site of the femur is lightly scarified with a chisel, to facilitate more rapid consolidation.

The trochanter is then temporarily transfixed to the femur with two thin Kirschner wires (which are later removed) and its new position checked with image-control. For this purpose the following method has proven itself to be of value: after drawing both limbs together evenly, a long Kirschner wire, which shows up plainly in the image control, is placed horizontally, parallel to both anterior superior spines, crossing the femoral head. The tip of the greater trochanter should be level with the center of the femoral head and its distance to the centre of the head should correspond to 2–2.5 times the radius of the femoral head.

The firm fixation of the greater trochanter is best executed with two lag screws, each equipped with a washer, inserted through previously bared bone (to avoid muscle necrosis) just distal to the origin of the gluteus medius, in a similar direction as the gluteal fibers, i.e. downward and medially. The direction of the lag screws counteracts the pelvitrochanteric muscle pull. The washers' increased surface area assures the firm fixation of the greater trochanter to its new site with no local mechanical irritation, allowing early exercizing of the limbs.

Fixation of the greater trochanter can also be accomplished with two heavy Kirschner wires inserted medially and upward. Through the direction of these wires, the resultant force of the abductors' pull creates a pressure of the greater trochanter on to the outside surface of the femur. However, the fixation with the screws is more stable (Fig. 17).

To achieve an even more reliable fastening of the greater trochanter, there must be performed, in addition to the metal fixation, a strongly braided suture line, securing the detached origin of the vastus lateralis to the insertion of the

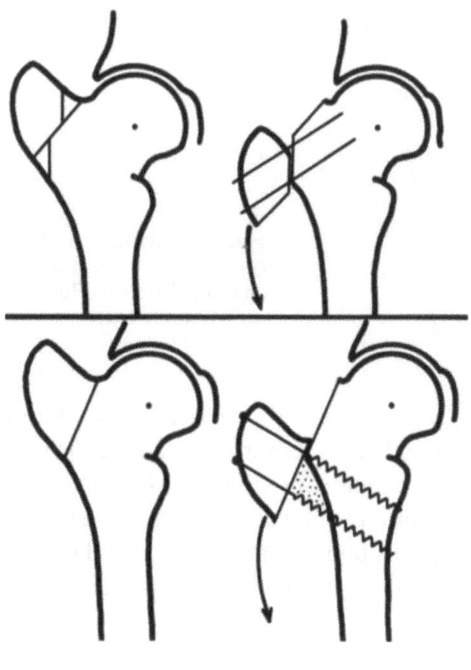

Fig. 17. Displacement osteotomy of the greater trochanter (for detailed description see text)

gluteus medius – strong enough in itself to absorb the pull of the pelvitrochanteric musculature and prevent the pulling-off of the greater trochanter (tension-band suture).

The above-described fixation is so dependable as to permit these patients to ambulate 24 h postoperatively, with the aid of crutches. However, an active exercise regime with active contractions of the pelvifemoral muscles is only possible after 3 weeks. Until then, these patients should not sit upright because in this position, the gluteus medius exerts a strong rotatory action on the trochanter, twisting it from its anchorage.

C. Lengthening of the Trochanter

In femoral neck shortening without "heightening" of the greater trochanter, where only the distance between the tip of the trochanter and the center of the femoral head has decreased, the lever arm of the pelvitrochanteric musculature can be lengthened (restored) by lateralization of the greater trochanter. In this case the greater trochanter is shifted laterally, and in the case of anteversion also ventrally, so that a wide cleft appears between the trochanter and the lateral femoral surface. The trochanter position is maintained by two wide-threaded

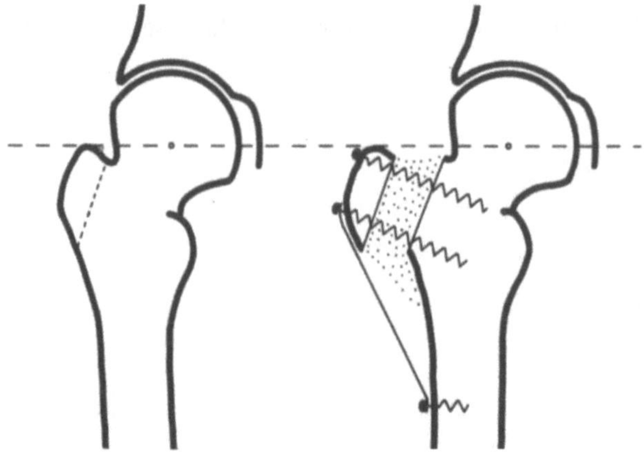

Fig. 18. Elongation osteotomy of the greater trochanter (for detailed description see text)

screws which are inserted horizontally as "positioning" screws, i.e., the screw threads grip equally well in the trochanter and in the femur, maintaining the cleft between them. To further secure fixation, a tight wire-suture is stretched from the neck of each of the screws distally to another small screw in the femur. The open cleft is filled with autogenous cancellous bone grafts. Lastly, for the same reasons mentioned above, the vastus lateralis is firmly sutured to the gluteus medius (Fig. 18).

D. The Intertrochanteric Double Osteotomy

When in the deformity of the proximal femoral end the malposition of the greater trochanter is accompanied by a short femoral neck and an incongruity of the hip joint surface, the trochanter transplantation alone is insufficient. With such multiple deformities a more extensive correction is necessary via the double osteotomy.

The principle of this operation is that through two more or less horizontal osteotomies at the level of (1) the upper edge and (2) the lower edge of the femoral neck, three fragments are created, each of which can independently be brought into its corrected position (Figs. 19, 20).

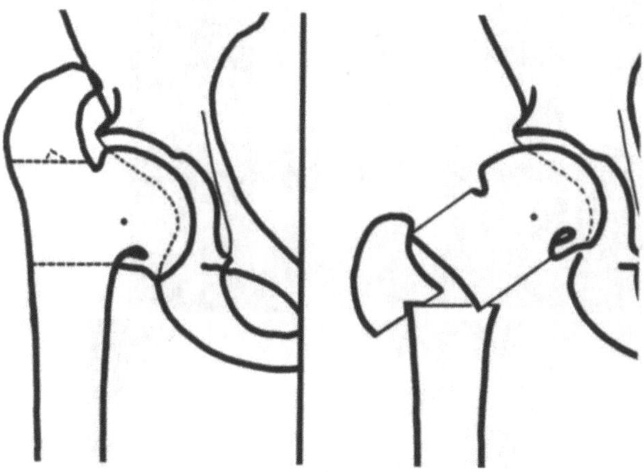

Fig. 19. Intertrochanteric double osteotomy. Two osteotomy cuts at the level of the upper and lower edge of the femoral neck divide the proximal end of the femur into three fragments, each of which can independently be brought into corrected position

As a first step, a Steinmann pin is inserted into the axis of the femoral neck, following which the two osteotomies are executed. The femoral neck fragment is redirected into the required position and moved medially in relation to the distal femoral fragment and the distal fragment is moved laterally so that the medial cortex of the distal fragment acts as a buttress to the lower corner of the femoral neck. The femoral neck now becomes longer. The mobilized trochanter is now transplanted distally and laterally and transfixed.

The osteosynthesis, in this relatively complicated osteotomy is performed variably, in accordance with the anatomic conditions encountered. The greater trochanter and femoral neck can both be passed over the long blade of a right-angle plate and placed under pressure with the distal fragment by means of a Müller jig. It is also possible to produce stabilization between the femoral neck and distal fragment, using a 130° plate and then screwing the greater trochanter and the other two fragments. Finally, as a third solution, it is possible to bring all three fragments into corrected position, fastening them temporarily together with Kirschner wires, then applying a moulded semitubular plate to the lateral aspect of the proximal femoral end. This plate is previously prepared using powerful shears to cut out a vertical slot from its proximal end to the first

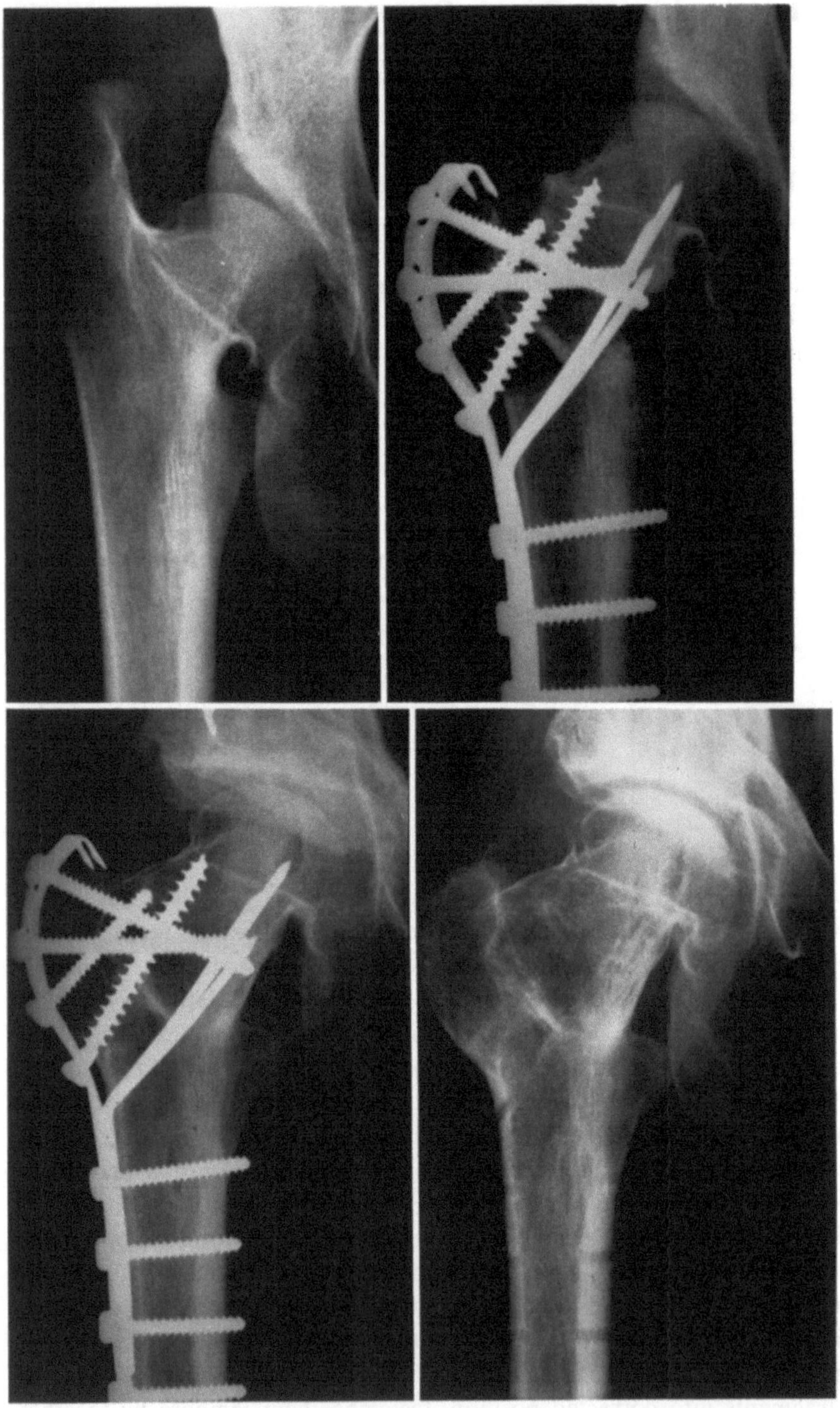

Fig. 20. Intertrochanteric double-osteotomy in a 16-year-old female at 3,9 and 18 months after surgery. The coverage of the femoral head has been accomplished by acetabular osteotomy

screw hole, thereby bifurcating it. After further trimming their tips to sharp points, the bifurcated limbs are bent inwardly to form hooks, which are inserted into the tip of the trochanter. With a clamp, the upper end is forced, like a hook, into the bone as additional anchorage. A diagonally inserted Kirschner wire gives assurance against shifting of the contact point of the femoral neck fragment on the underlying buttress of the shaft's medial corticalis; then all the screws are firmly applied. The remaining spaces between fragments are packed with cancellous bone grafts. This described osteosynthesis is performed so securely as to even render it for immediate motion therapy. Bone healing occurs quickly afterwards, permitting full weight-bearing in 12 weeks. After 2 years, structural remodelling is so advanced as to render the original osteotomy surfaces unrecognizable.

Conclusion

A review has been given of the modern treatment for correction of deformities of the upper end of the femur encountered in congenital hip dysplasia. The departure from former methods of treatment has been justified by the much improved results obtained. These improved biomechanical results have been maintained, clinically and radiologically, after an appreciable time interval.

References

Allgöwer, M., Kinzl, L., Matter, P., Perren, S. M., Rüedi, T: Die dynamische Kompressionsplatte. Berlin–Heidelberg–New York: Springer 1973

Müller, M. E.: Die hüftnahen Femurosteotomien. 2nd edition. Stuttgart: Thieme 1971

Müller, M. E., Allgöwer, M., Willenegger, H.: Manual der Osteosynthese, 2. Aufl. Berlin–Heidelberg–New York: Springer 1977

Wagner, H.: Principien der Korrekturosteotomie am Bein. Orthopäde **6,** 145–177 (1977)

Our Experience with Salter's Innominate Osteotomy in the Treatment of Hip Dysplasia

E. Morscher*

Generally speaking, the main problem in the treatment of hip dysplasia is not reduction of a dislocated hip, but stabilization of the achieved reduction. In 1961, Salter described an innominate osteotomy, which now bears his name, for improved stabilization of the hip joint in the treatment of dislocation and subluxation. The principle of this operation is that following an osteotomy of the pelvis in the linea innominata, the inferior portion of the pelvis, i.e., the entire acetabulum including pubic bone and ischium, be tilted anterolaterally and caudally, using the symphysis as the fulcrum (Fig. 1). As a result, the acetabulum is shifted downward from its former, anterolaterally directed position. Apart from this acetabular maldirection, Salter considers capsular elongation and contractures of the adductors and iliopsoas muscles to be the main causes of the instability (Salter and Dubos, 1974).

Salter considers the main indications for his operation to be either the primary treatment of dislocations and subluxations of the hip in children aged 18 months to 6 years, i.e., for cases that are discovered late, or where normalization of the hip joint by conservative means can no longer be expected. Further indications for innominate osteotomy are primary operations – without previous treatment – of congenital subluxations from the age of $1^1/_2$ years into adulthood, secondary operations of residual dislocations between $1^1/_2$ and 6 years, and residual subluxations in cases of failure of previous treatment from $1^1/_2$ years to adulthood.

The necessity for acetabuloplasties actually is present only when the diagnosis of hip dysplasia has been made too late. Studies at our institution (Jani, 1976) show that normalization of a dysplastic acetabulum is still successful in 96% of the cases where reduction or initial treatment is undertaken before the age of 1 year. If reduction is performed between the ages of 1 and 2, acetabular normalization occurs only in 55% of the patients; after the second year of life, in only 20% of the cases.

* Orthopaedic Department, University of Basel, Basel, Switzerland

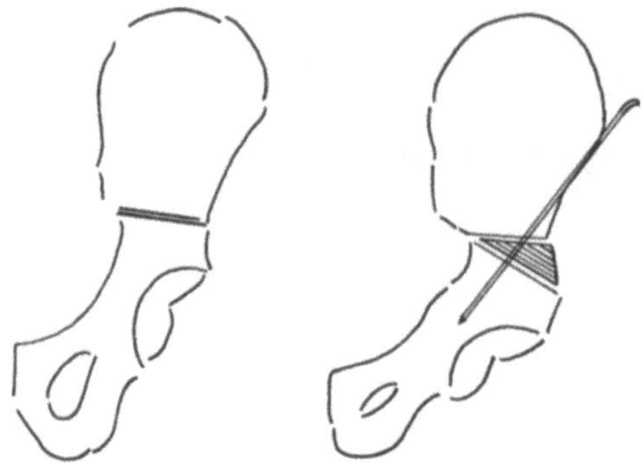

Fig. 1. Diagrammatic representation of innominate osteotomy of SALTER. (a) Left pelvis, osteotomy along the innominate line drawn in. (b) State after osteotomy: the inferior portion of the pelvis is displaced ventrolaterally; the position is fixed by a bone wedge inserted in the osteotomy gap and by a KIRSCHNER wire piercing both fragments and the bone chip

The results of the formerly widely performed *extracapsular shelf operations,* in which the existing acetabular roof is simply folded down or enlarged by insertion of a bone chip, did not prove satisfactory. These methods are mainly linked with the names of Spitzy, Gill, Lance, et al.

The various acetabuloplasties are incomplete pelvic osteotomies, where the acetabular roof is levered down and the resulting gap is filled with bone chips, thus supporting the newly created acetabular roof. Of the different methods (Albee, Wiberg, Pemberton), that of Pemberton is surely the most extensive and effective. With respect to acetabuloplasty, Salter is concerned about the rise in pressure in the joint due to folding down the acetabular roof and the incongruity of the acetabulum that follows bending in the Y-line.

Important aspects in the operative treatment of dysplastic acetabula were revealed by the *pelvic osteotomy of* Chiari (1955). Not only can the hip joint be well stabilized, but the possible lateral position of the femoral head can also be eliminated, if after osteotomy of the ilium, the head of the femur is displaced medially, together with the dysplastic acetabulum. In addition, this operation acts favorably on the weight-bearing capability of the joint since not only is the area of loading shortened by the medial displacement but the muscular lever arm is also elongated, as Chiari himself demonstrated (1974). A disadvantage of the method – particularly in regard and in contrast to the operation of Salter to be discussed here – is the fact that the pressure-receiving area is formed by the joint capsule that is interposed between the femoral head and the newly formed acetabular roof. Through compressive strain, this capsular tissue may well be transformed into fibrous cartilage, but it is qualitatively undoubtedly inferior to hyaline cartilage.

In all those cases where a pathologically increased neck-shaft angle and increased antetorsion angle threaten the stability of the hip joint, the *intertrochanteric varus correction and derotation osteotomy of the proximal femur* has become almost a routine procedure in Europe, both as sole operation and in combination with acetabuloplasty. In 1973 Weber evaluated 315 operations on the acetabular roofs of 254 patients in connection with the Swiss multicenter study on the treatment of congenital dislocation of the hip: innominate osteotomy had been combined with detorsion-varus osteotomy at the proximal end of the femur in 66%, with acetabuloplasty in 73.4%, and with a Chiari medial displacement osteotomy even in 87.7% of the cases.

Although detorsion-varus osteotomy by itself, i.e., without other operations on the acetabulum, produced essential advantages in the treatment of dislocated hips, it became apparent that initial exceptions regarding this type of osteotomy were too optimistic. In many cases, the desired adaption and molding of the acetabulum to the newly created anatomic and joint-mechanical conditions did not materialize. Our own patient population and that of the Swiss multicenter study on 1361 dislocated hips revealed that acetabular normalization by means of this operation alone was achieved in only 20% of the cases. However, it ought to be mentioned that the intertrochanteric derotation-varus osteotomy had rarely been carried out before the second and, in most cases, even after the fourth year of life. Also, the almost routine straightening of the femoral neck prevented definitive stabilization of the hip joint in many cases.

As mentioned, the principle of Salter's innominate osteotomy is an anterolateral and caudal rotation of the whole acetabulum together with the pubic and ischial bones, whereby, contrary to acetabuloplasties, the symphysis is the pivot and not the Y-line. Thus, the acetabular roof is not simply levered down, but the whole acetabulum is brought into a more favorable position for stability of the joint. The aperture of the acetabulum no longer faces anterolaterally, but rather more caudally; in this way, the head of the femur is provided with a considerably better roof. The weight-bearing area is enlarged, and therefore the total stress on the joint is distributed. But despite providing a better roof over the femoral head, the total pressure on the joint is increased by innominate osteotomy. If the position of the acetabulum is studied with an X-ray tracing before and after osteotomy, it is obvious that it has not only changed its direction, but that the whole acetabulum has also been displaced caudally (Fig. 1). This caudal displacement – Utterback and MacEwen (1974) call it the "long leg effect" – arises from the spreading effect of the osteotomy, where the inferior fragment has to be pushed anterolaterally and, most importantly, also caudally. The consequence is that the head of the femur is also pushed caudally together with the acetabulum, and a rise in pressure develops in the joint.

The increase in tension, which frequently still exists after a period of preoperative extension therapy and which is manifest in, among other things, contractures of the adductors and iliopsoas muscles, reduces the stability of the hip especially when weight is applied; for this reason, Salter advises release of these muscles.

The tension and raised pressure, adversely affecting articular function and blood supply of the head of the femur, can be avoided by simultaneous varus correction of the neck of the femur; thus, the reorientation of the acetabulum can be performed with greater ease and effectiveness. This operation likewise effects considerable release of the adductors and iliopsoas muscles, and they need not be divided.

As follows from these comments and as demonstrated in Table 1, there is no *one* operation as yet available which corrects all deformities and malpositions of

Table 1. Effects of different "hip-stabilizing" operations[a]

	Desired	Extracapsular shelf operation	Acetabuloplasty	Medial displacement osteotomy of the pelvis (CHIARI)	Derotation and varus-osteotomy	SALTER innominate osteotomy
Head of femur	Medial displacement	0	0	++	+	(−)
Weight-bearing area	Enlarged	+	+	+	(+)	+
	Formed of hyaline acetabular cartilage	− −	+	− −	(+)	++
Total pressure in joint	Reduced	0	−	(+)	+	−
Muscular lever arm	Elongated	0	0	+	+	0
Weight arm	Shortened	0	0	+	+	(−)
Proximal end of femur	Varus-corrected and derotated	0	0	0	++	0

[a] +, favorable effect. 0, no effect. −, unfavorable effect. In parentheses: inconstant or insignificant effect

the dysplastic joint, which has no intrinsic disadvantage, and which could be regarded as a universal solution for the improved stability of dislocated hips. One or another single surgical method may be satisfactory in individual cases, but this is true only infrequently in our experience. For the majority of cases, therefore, it appears expedient to combine a pelvic operation with varus correction and detorsion of the neck of the femur. Unfavorable acetabular conditions and pathologic axis deviations at the proximal femur can thus be corrected. We believe that the combination of an innominate osteotomy with a corrective osteotomy of the proximal end of the femur is indicated above all in cases of children beyond the age of 4 years. Based on the theoretical considerations discussed, we formerly combined these two operations almost routinely. Today, as a rule we omit the derotation-varus correction osteotomy in children under age 4, if the head of the femur is not displaced laterally and there is no subluxation (Figs. 2 and 3). However, spontaneous self-correction of faulty angular conditions at the proximal end of the femur following innominate osteotomy is not, as Salter claims, the rule, but depends essentially on the age of the children. According to our experience, this correction may be anticipated in younger children as mentioned, but hardly after age 4. The advisability of a concomitant osteotomy of the femur in "older children" is supported by our experience of severe structural changes of the femoral head in a 6-year-old patient on whom only an innominate osteotomy had been performed. Among Salter's own patients (Salter and Dubos, 1974), the rate of femoral head necrosis was 5.7% for combined open reduction and innominate osteotomy. In the group of residual dislocations and residual subluxation following unsuccessful previous treatment, it was 30%!

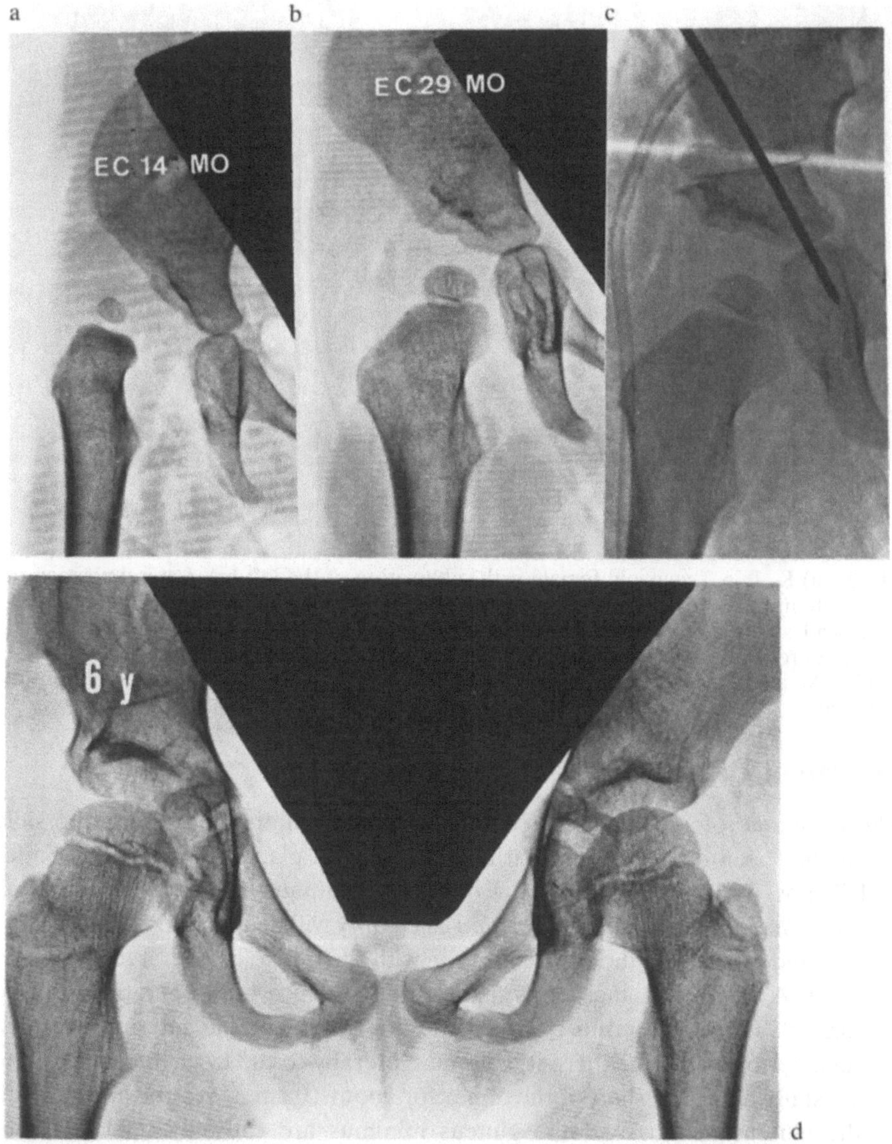

Fig. 2. (a) *EC*, a 14-month-old female with a congenital dislocation of the hip. (b) State after overhead extension, closed reduction, and aftertreatment in a Denis Browne abduction splint. (c) Innominate osteotomy at the age of $2^1/_2$ years. (d) State at checkup at the age of 6 years: largely physiologic conditions of hip joint

In the Swiss multicenter study on results of treatments for congenital hip dislocations, Weber (1973) found structural disorders of the hip following 14.9% of 49 Salter osteotomies, mainly in those cases without simultaneous derotation-varus osteotomy. The rate of structural disorders of the head was comparably high in acetabuloplasties (15.4%), whereas after pelvic osteotomy of Chiari it amounted to only 1%!

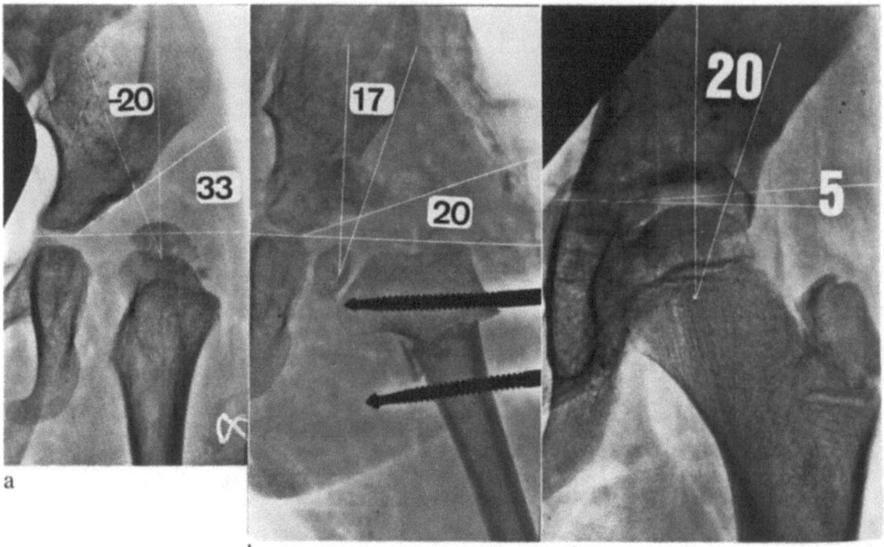

Fig. 3. (a) K. J., a 3-year-old female with subluxation of the left hip. Lateral position of head of femur. CE angle = −20°, Ac angle = 33°. (b) State after innominate osteotomy and simultaneous detorsion-varus correction osteotomy. The femoral head was well-centered due to the osteotomy at the proximal end of the femur: CE angle = +17°, Ac angle = 20°. (c) Checkup 7 years postoperatively: physiologic conditions at hip joint

Operation Technique

The technique of innominate osteotomy, including hints for avoiding possible errors, has been described in great detail in several places (Salter, 1961; Salter and Dubos, 1974). Therefore, only our own technique of *combined operation according to Salter with varus-derotation osteotomy* will be described here.

The child is placed in the supine position with the side to be operated on slightly elevated. A single skin incision is made through which both operations can be performed. The incision runs from the anterior quarter of the anterior iliac crest to the anterior iliac spine; here it continues laterally to the trochanter major and then distally along the shaft of the femur for about 10 cm. Next, the anterior half of the gluteus medius and the gluteus minimus are carefully detached subperiosteally from the pelvic crest and the wing of ilium down to the capsule of the hip joint. The detached musculature is retracted by means of a Hohmann (Blount) retractor introduced into the greater ischiadic foramen. After this, the musculature on the inner aspect of the ilium is detached, also strictly subperiosteally, by proceeding with a periosteal elevator from the area between anterior superior and inferior iliac spine to the greater sciatic notch. If open reduction is necessary at the same time, it is easily achieved by a ventrocranial incision into the capsule. The osteotomy is linear from the greater sciatic notch to the anterior inferior iliac spine.

Salter recommends that the bone graft required for supporting the osteotomy be obtained from the anterior portion of the iliac wing. However, since the apophysis of the iliac crest is still very wide in small children and removal of a bone graft from this area could result in growth disturbance of the ilium, we dispense with the use of an autologous bone graft and insert bank bone. This makes it possible to use a broader graft and thus also minimizes the risk of its tilting. Since, as mentioned, the head of the femur has to be pushed downward on spreading the osteotomy site, the varus correction-derotation osteotomy is carried out *prior* to inserting the bone graft into the osteotomy.

The fascia lata is incised in the direction of its longitudinal fibers from the trochanter major in the caudal portion of the skin incision. The lateral vastus muscle is detached from the shaft of the femur at its insertion; the intertrochanteric region is exposed subperiosteally and retracted by means of Hohmann (Blount) retractors. Through a stab incision made dorsal to the skin incision a Schanz screw is introduced laterally, distal to the epiphyseal plate of the greater trochanter, exactly along the axis of the neck of the femur. A Steinmann pin is drilled into the shaft of the femur approximately 3–4 cm below the Schanz screw, corresponding to the desired varus correction and derotation of the femoral neck. It is assumed that the degree of the desired detorsion and varus correction of the neck of the femur has previously been determined by special roentgenograms.

The osteotomy can now be carried out parallel to the Schanz screw. Next, a bony wedge with a medial base is obtained from the distal fragment in such a fashion that the osteotomy areas lie parallel to the Steinmann pin at this fragment. This is followed by a concomitant torsion and tilting of the fragments till the Schanz screw and the Steinmann pin lie parallel and in the same plane. The distal fragment is slightly displaced medially in order to prevent overstraining of the medial condyle at the knee and to reduce the bending stress at the neck of the femur. The Steinmann pin is then replaced by a Schanz screw, which is likewise introduced through a separate stab incision dorsal to the skin incision. Two "fixateurs externes" are now applied to the screw, allowing compression of the osteotomy for better stabilization.

The Salter operation is concluded only at the end of the varus-detorsion osteotomy! The osteotomy site is spread with towel clips that grip both pelvic fragments firmly, and the inferior fragment is strongly pulled anterocaudally and laterally. The bone wedge is now inserted into the osteotomy. For stabilization of the fragments and the bone graft wedged between them, a Kirschner wire is inserted from the upper fragment through the bone chip into the lower fragment.

Postoperatively, a plaster of Paris hip spica is applied and left for six weeks. Thereafter, the spica cast, Schanz screws and Kirschner wire are removed, and mobilization is commenced.

Results

Our own experience with Salter's innominate osteotomy derives from 69 operations, performed between 1963 and 1976. The operation was combined 32 times with a derotation-varus correction osteotomy at the proximal end of the femur; as a single procedure, it was performed 37 times. Our results and experiences are based on two separate reevaluations:

The first, very small group comprised 13 children, with 15 hips on which a Salter osteotomy had been carried out in the years 1963 and 1964. These patients were carefully examined and radiographed, first in 1965 and again in 1973 (Morscher, 1965, 1973, 1974).

The second group was assessed in conjunction with the first in order to compare innominate osteotomy with acetabuloplasty and Chiari's osteotomy (Jani, 1976). It included 121 acetabuloplasties, carried out between 1963 and 1974. There were 49 innominate osteotomies, 36 acetabuloplasties, and 36 pelvic osteotomies using Chiari's method.

In evaluating each method for stabilization of the hip joint in the treatment of dysplasia, subluxation or dislocation, the roentgenogram is of crucial significance.

One of the most important and reliable criteria for the roof over the head of the femur is the CE angle of Wiberg (Wiberg, 1939). According to measurements by Severin (1943), values above 20° are considered normal in children between 6 and 13 years, values between 15° and 20° are problematic, and those below 15° are certainly pathologic.

Another important criterion for stability of the hip joint is the Ac or acetabular roof angle of Hilgenreiner (1939). When measuring this angle, one must remember that it can vary quite considerably according to the inclination of the pelvis. Faber (1938) recorded average values of 15° for healthy hip joints of 3–4-year-old children.

Results in the First Group

The average age of the children was 3.9 years (minimum: 1 year, 8 months; maximum: 7 years, 4 months) at the time of operation on the 15 hip joints. The mean time of observation was 7.8 years (minimum: 5 years, 2 months; maximum: 9 years, 4 months).

The CE angle was preoperatively pathologic in all cases and ranged from −24° to +14°; the mean was +2.1°. It improved postoperatively to 20.5° (0°–35°). Mean values registered at checkups were 26.8° (0°–38°) (Fig. 4a).

The acetabular angle was improved from an average of 34.8° (21°–51°) to 23.7° (13°–42°) postoperatively. The subsequently observed further improvement of the acetabular roof was even more pleasing than that of the CE angle and attained on the average 12.5° (3°–37°) (Fig. 4b).

Altogether, 11 of 15 operated hip joints in this first group became practically completely normal, both in regard to conditions at the acetabulum and the proximal end of the femur. Two hips were scored "satisfactory to good" because the femoral neck reverted to a valgus position. Two cases remained unsatisfactory; in one, a Chiari pelvic osteotomy has since been performed with good results.

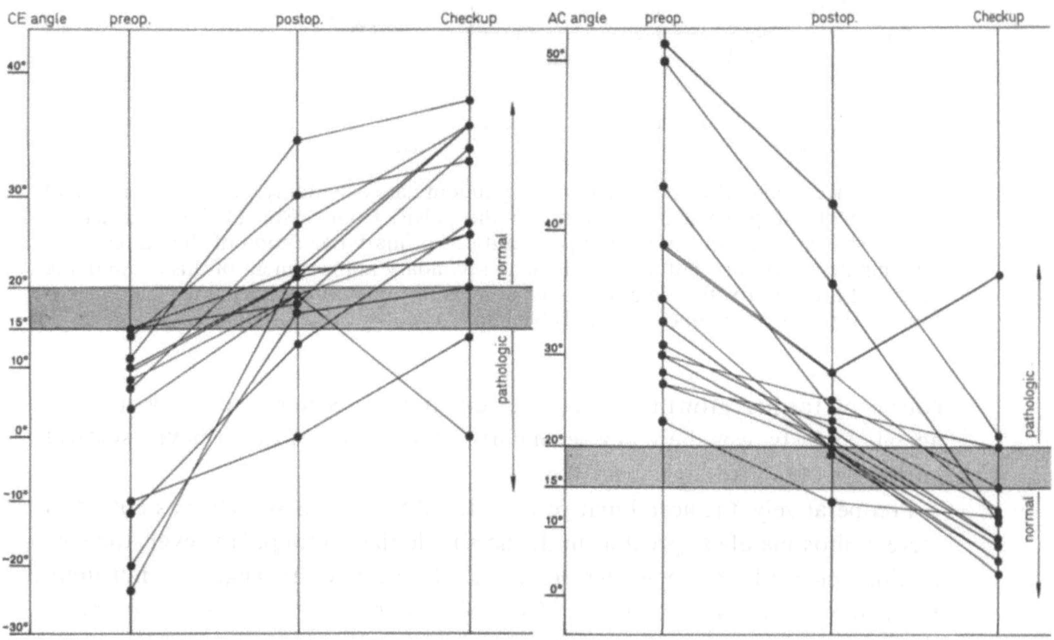

Fig. 4. Change in the *CE* angle of Wiberg (a), and acetabular *(Ac)* angle (b) following innominate osteotomy of SALTER (with and without detorsion-varus osteotomy). The values of the angle refer to the state before and immediately after operation, and at checkup (on average, 7.8 years postoperatively)

Results in the Second Group

In the second group, where 121 acetabuloplasties were reexamined, our primary intention was to compare the three types of operations for stabilization of a dysplastic hip performed at our institution in order to improve differentiation of the indications for the individual techniques (Jani, 1974, 1976) (Figs. 5 a–c).

The preoperative Ac angle averaged 40° in the 49 innominate osteotomies. Correction of this angle by 12°, i.e., from 40° to 28°, was achieved by the operation. Subsequently, further improvement of this angle occurred. On the average, it was 20° five years postoperatively (Fig. 3 a).

Among the 36 acetabuloplasties, the preoperative Ac angle was greater than in the patients operated on using Salter's method. Better primary correction was achieved by acetabuloplasties. In practically all cases, the acetabuloplasty had been combined with a derotation-varus correction osteotomy of the proximal end of the femur. As with the Salter osteotomy, the Ac angle improved in the

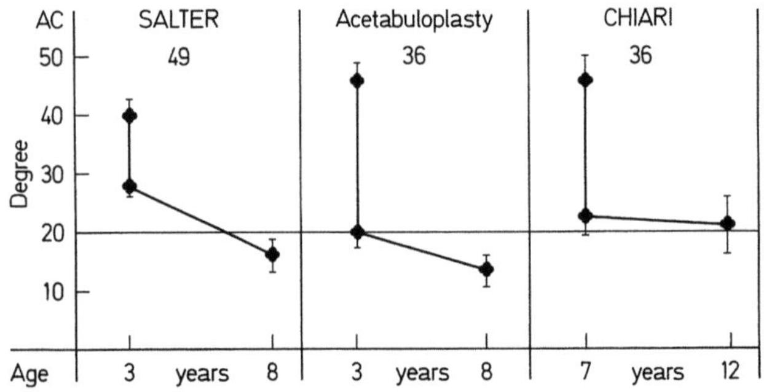

Fig. 5. Correction of the acetabular angle by innominate osteotomy, acetabuloplasty, and Chiari medial displacement osteotomy of the pelvis. Comparison of the three curves clearly shows the relatively limited possibility of primary correction of the Ac angle in innominate osteotomy, but a very adequate secondary improvement of this angle in the course of further growth — a development almost completely absent in the Chiari osteotomy. (Abscissa: age at operation and checkup)

course of further growth. In no case, either after Salter osteotomy or after acetabuloplasty, was there any secondary deterioration of the achieved surgical correction of the Ac angle (Fig. 3b).

Preoperatively, the acetabular roof angles of the 36 Chiari pelvic osteotomies were approximately as great as in the acetabuloplasty group. However, the correction achieved was somewhat less: Usually the normal range was not quite reached by the Chiari osteotomy. Moreover, contrary to the two other methods, the Ac angle did not improve during further growth, and in a few cases, deteriorations were observed, compared with immediate postoperative measurements (Fig. 3c)!

Discussion and Conclusions

In comparison with other methods, particularly the acetabuloplasty and pelvic osteotomy of Chiari, our experience with the innominate osteotomy of Salter has shown that it is an excellent procedure for creating normal physiologic hip conditions in a dysplastic hip, provided that the indication is proper. The explanation lies in the fact that the whole acetabulum is tilted around a pivot in the symphysis; thus the weight-bearing area between the head of the femur and acetabulum is formed and enlarged by hyaline articular cartilage. Analyses of individual cases show that a disadvantage of innominate osteotomy is the limitation of primary correction possible during performance of the operation. Undoubtedly, this limitation is essentially due to counterpressure exerted by the head of the femur against the caudal displacement of the acetabulum during operation. Our reevaluations also show that the average improvement of the Ac angle was only 6° in the four cases of the first group, where the Salter osteotomy had been performed without simultaneous varus correction of the neck of the femur, whereas it was nearly twice as much (11°) in the other cases in which combined procedures had been adopted.

In the second group, the Ac angle improved by an average of 12°. In this respect, our results agree with those of Utterback and MacEwen (1974), who observed 10° average improvement in acetabular index. Therefore, Chapchal (1974) considers innominate osteotomy to be indicated in dysplastic hips with an Ac angle of maximally 30°. But the fact that considerable further improvement may be expected in the course of growth justifies performing the operation even in severe cases, especially if it is combined with a detorsion-varus osteotomy (Fig. 6).

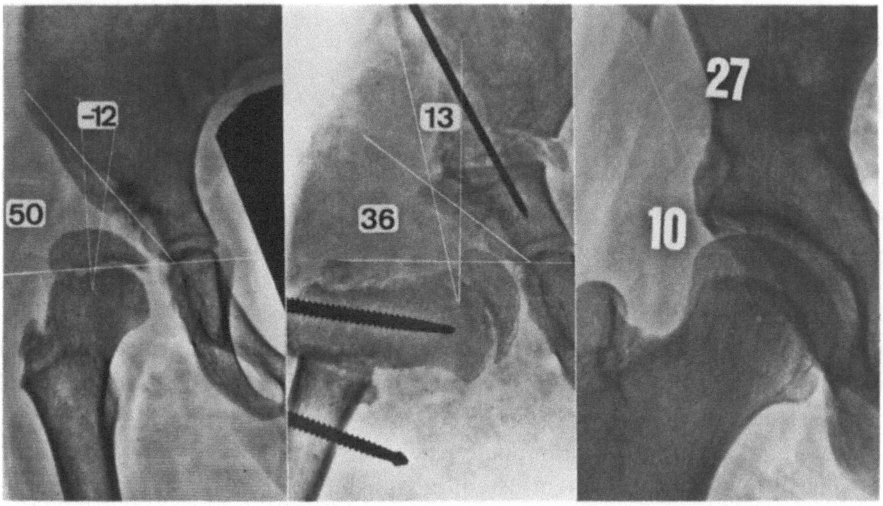

a b c

Fig. 6. (a) St. M., a $5^1/_2$-year-old female with residual subluxation of the right hip, CE angle = −12°, Ac angle = 50° (!). Despite the very steep acetabular roof, innominate osteotomy was performed, but with simultaneous rotation and varus correction of the femoral neck. The CE angle was corrected by 15° to 13°, the Ac angle by 14° to only 36°. In the course of growth, considerable further improvement of both angle values took place so that normal values were measured $8^1/_2$ years postoperatively at the age of $14^1/_2$. (CE angle = 27°, Ac angle = 10°). The minor deformity of the head of the femur (head-neck position of the epiphysis) was already present before the operation

One would expect greater corrections of the Ac angle to be achieved in younger children since tilting in the symphysis pubis is not so easily accomplished in older children. However, in the age groups that we examined, no such age dependence was noted.

Thus, today we consider innominate osteotomy indicated mainly in dysplasia of the hip joint with a pathologic Ac angle up to around 40° in children between 2 and 4 or at most 6 years of age. If the acetabular angle is above 40°, we prefer an acetabuloplasty for patients up to 5 years of age. For patients above 6 years, we consider Chiari's medial displacement osteotomy of the pelvis to be the most suitable procedure.

Since with increasing age, spontaneous corrections at the proximal femur decline and moreover, especially in children over the age of 4 years, joint pressure and adductor and iliopsoas tension increase during innominate osteotomy, we combine this procedure with detorsion-varus osteotomy, particularly in cases of children over age 4.

Comparison of innominate osteotomy with acetabuloplasty and pelvic osteotomy of Chiari resulted in a clarification of their specific indications. There is no doubt that these three procedures are not competitive but rather mutually complementary means toward the improved stabilization of a dysplastic hip. No method by itself can produce optimal results in every case.

Summary

Two evaluations were carried out at the Basel University Orthopaedic Hospital comparing one group of 15 hips operated on using innominate osteotomy with a second group of 121 acetabular plasties (49 innominate osteotomies, 36 acetabuloplasties, and 36 Chiari pelvic osteotomies). Based on these, an attempt was made to improve definition of the specific indications for innominate osteotomy, for no method exists which is capable of correcting every malformation and malposition encountered in dysplastic hips at different ages with an equal degree of success.

The great advantage of innominate osteotomy – especially when compared to Chiari's medial displacement osteotomy of the pelvis – is that a congruous acetabular roof is formed largely by its own hyaline cartilage, which has an optimal load-bearing capacity.

The disadvantages of the operation – the rise in pressure within the joint and the irremediableness of an existing lateral position of the head of the femur – can be eliminated by a detorsion-varus osteotomy of the proximal end of the femur performed simultaneously with innominate osteotomy. Although the possibility of primary correction of the acetabular angle is much smaller in innominate osteotomy than in both other methods, it is equalized in great measure by the regularly observed secondary improvement of the Ac angle in the course of further growth.

References

Chapchal, G.: Indications for the Various Types of Pelvic Osteotomy. Clin. Orthop. **98,** 111–115 (1974)

Chiari, K.: Ergebnisse mit der Beckenosteotomie als Pfannendachplastik. Z. Orthop. **87,** 14–26 (1955)

Chiari, K.: Medial Displacement Osteotomy of the Pelvis. Clin. Orthop. **98,** 55–71 (1974)

Faber, A.: Das Röntgenbild des Hüftgelenks beim Säugling und zur Pathologie der angeborenen Dysplasie des Hüftgelenks. Verh. Dtsch. Orthop. Ges. **32.** Kongr. 251–272 (1938)
Hilgenreiner, H.: Ein sicheres Verfahren zur Diagnose der angeborenen Hüftgelenksverrenkung. Z. Orthop. **69,** 488–490 (1939)
Jani, L.: Entwicklung der dysplastischen Hüftgelenkspfanne nach der Overhead-Extension. Orthop. Praxis **9,** 365–369 (1973)
Jani, L.: Die operative Behandlung der praearthrotischen Deformitäten der Hüftgelenkspfanne bei der kongenitalen Hüftluxation. Z. Orthop. **112,** 605–609 (1974)
Jani, L.: Differenzierte Indikationsstellung zu den verschiedenen pfannendachplastischen Eingriffen. Tagung 76 der Ges. für Orthopädie der DDR, Magdeburg 1976
Morscher, E.: Kombinierte Beckenosteotomie nach SALTER mit varisierender Detorsionsosteotomie am oberen Femurende. In CHAPCHAL: Beckenosteotomie-Pfannendachplastik. **78–86,** Thieme, Stuttgart: 1965
Morscher, E.: Die Beckenosteotomie nach SALTER in der Behandlung der dysplastischen Hüftgelenkspfanne. Orthopäde **2,** 250–252 (1973)
Morscher, E.: Erfahrungen mit der Beckenosteotomie nach SALTER. Orthop. Praxis **10,** 11–15 (1974)
Salter, R. B.: Innominate osteotomy in the treatment of congenital dislocation and subluxation of the hip. J. Bone Jt. Surg. **43-B,** 518–539 (1961)
Salter, R. B., Dubos, J. P.: The first fifteen years' personal experience with innominate osteotomy in the tratment of congenital dislocation and subluxation of the hip. Clin. Orthop. **98,** 72–103 (1974)
Severin, F.: Spätresultate unblutiger Behandlung von Luxatio coxae congenita. Z. Orthop. **74,** 52–75 (1943)
Utterback, T. D., Mac Ewen, G. D.: Comparison of pelvic osteotomies for the surgical correction of the conenital hip. Clin. Orthop. **98,** 104–110 (1974)
Weber, A.: Beckenosteotomie und Acetabuloplastik in der Behandlung der residuellen Hüftdysplasie. Jahreskongreß der Schweiz. Ges. für Orthopädie 1973
Wiberg, G.: Studies on dysplastic acetabular and congenital subluxation of the hip joint. Acta chir. scand. **83,** suppl. (1939)

Revised and updated English translation from the German edition *Der Orthopäde,* Vol. 2, pp. 250–252 (1973),

Chiari Pelvic Osteotomy for Hip Dysplasia in Patients Below the Age of 20

H. J. Strauß*

In the formation and function of the human hip joint the roof of the acetabulum is very important. Incongruity between the acetabulum and the head of femur will lead to altered mechanics with subsequent abnormal development in children and secondary osteoarthritis in adults.

Treatment of hip dysplasia is best undertaken during early infancy, where conservative treatment is utilized during the first few months of life. Pathologic weight-bearing of a dysplastic acetabulum can only partly be corrected by osteotomies of the femoral neck. Therefore, several techniques have been devised which redirect the acetabulum. The different methods of acetabuloplasty and the innominate osteotomy of Salter have limited application. By contrast, the pelvic osteotomy of Chiari, first described in 1953, has proven valuable in many severe dysplasias.

Its principle is a transverse osteotomy of the pelvic isthmus at the level of the cranial insertion of the capsule with displacement of the fragments. This brings the hip joint pivot closer to the body axis. In this manner pressure on the joint is relieved, greater efficiency of the pelvitrochanteric musculature is achieved, the head of the femur receives an osseous support, and the interposed capsule is later transformed to fibrocartilage under functional stress (Fig. 1).

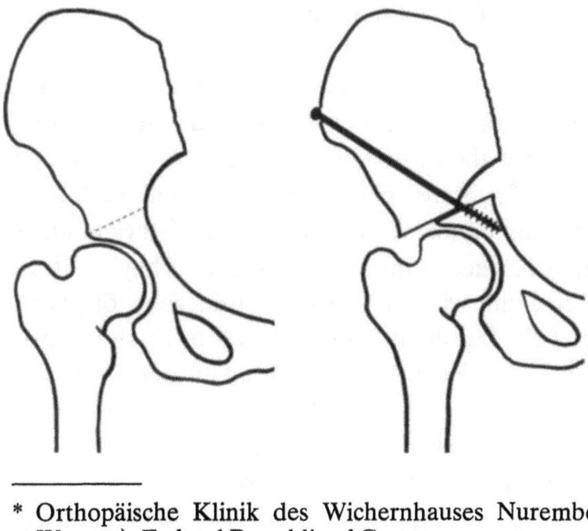

Fig. 1. Diagram of pelvic osteotomy with screw in place

* Orthopäische Klinik des Wichernhauses Nuremberg/Altdorf (Chief: Prof. Dr. H. Wagner), Federal Republic of Germany

We have reviewed our experience of the Chiari osteotomy from 1966 to 1976. At the Orthopädische Klinik des Wichernhauses in Altdorf we did 194 osteotomies on 156 patients during this period of time. 164 hips in 127 patients were available for follow-up examination. In 30, the osteotomy was bilateral; in 7, the osteotomy had to be repeated on the same side. Chiari's pelvic osteotomy was done in 141 cases of dysplasia with a CE angle of less than 10°. In 13 selected cases, it served to brace a reduced femoral head after severe dislocation. The youngest patient was 4 years old, the eldest 19 years, the average age was 13.02 years. Most of the patients were girls in a ratio of 3.4:1 (see Table 1).

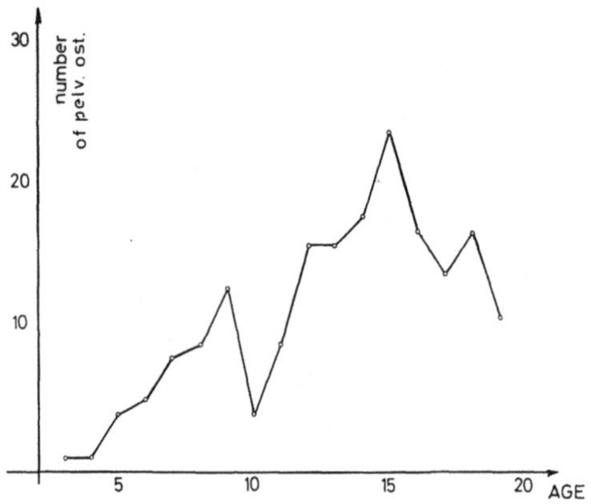

Table 1. Age and sex of patients on whom Chiari's pelvic osteotomy was performed
Sex:
female : male 3.4 : 1

For the operation an anterior approach to the hip was chosen, approaching the joint between sartorius muscle and tensor fasciae latae. The tensor fasciae latae together with a small portion of the gluteus medius was stripped subperiosteally off the wing of the ilium. In order to avoid too high an osteotomy, the capsular insertion at the pelvic wall has to be displaced distally since it often extends cranially for a considerable distance. After defining the level of the osteotomy on the X-ray image intensifier, elevators which conform to the shape of the bone are inserted medially and laterally around the pelvic isthmus into the greater sciatic foramen, for protection during the osteotomy which is carried out with a Gigli saw. Osteotomy with this saw has the advantage that splintering is avoided and displacement of the fragments is facilitated because of the smooth surface of the osteotomy. The fragments are manipulated until the head of the femur is completely covered by the proximal surface of the acetabular roof. They are fixed in this position with a screw or Kirschner wire. In cases of considerable displacement any postoperative shifting of the fragments can be prevented by interposition of a bone chip or a small strip of bone cement. Since we consider the avoidance of immobilization to be of decisive importance for satisfactory functional results, the limb is placed in a plastic splint. Movement is permitted after 24 hours, and walking with partial weight-bearing after two days.

The most common errors of pelvic osteotomy of Chiari are: the osteotomy being done too high thus leaving insufficient support for the craniolateral segment of the femoral head, or done too low, thus causing damage to the acetabular cartilage and joint capsule. Other mistakes are: failure to make the cut with a superior inclination from lateral to medial or inadequate displacement of the fragments. Under no circumstance should the osteotomy disturb the sacroiliac joint. Postoperative complications included hematomas in 12 cases, which were drained by aspiration or reexploration. Reexploration was necessary 5 times for infected hematoma. Peroneal paresis was observed in 3 cases which recovered rapidly and completely.

The following subsidiary operations were employed in addition to the pelvic osteotomy (Table 2).

Transposition of the greater trochanter was necessary in 67 cases because of high trochanteric position and insufficiency of the hip musculature. Intertrochanteric osteotomy had to be performed 71 times for correction of malposition of the femoral neck. In 4 cases of poliomyelitis, the iliopsoas tendon was transposed onto the greater trochanter at the time of the osteotomy.

In order to evaluate our results, clinical and roentgenologic findings before and after operation were compared. The period of observation ranged from 6 months to 10 years. In order to compare the functional efficiency of the Chiari osteotomy more precisely with the initial condition of the patients, they were divided into 4 groups according to the severity of the dysplasia, with subgroups according to the shape of the femoral head (Table 3).

Table 2. Operations complementary to osteotomy

A Transposition of the trochanter:	
at time of osteotomy	3
before osteotomy	38
after osteotomy	26
B Intertrochanteric osteotomy:	
at time of pelvic osteotomy	16
before pelvic osteotomy	43
after pelvic osteotomy	12
C Transposition of iliopsoas	
at time of pelvic osteotomy	4

Table 3. Classification of patients into 4 groups, with findings listed according to classification

Group I:	Slight dysplasia, femoral head coverage above 60%		43
	a) good contour of femoral head	21	
	b) deformity of femoral head	22	
Group II:	Moderate dysplasia, femoral head coverage between 50–60%		65
	a)	25	
	b)	40	
Group III:	Severe dysplasia, femoral coverage below 50%		43
	a)	12	
	b)	31	
Group IV:	Dislocations		13
	a)	5	
	b)	8	

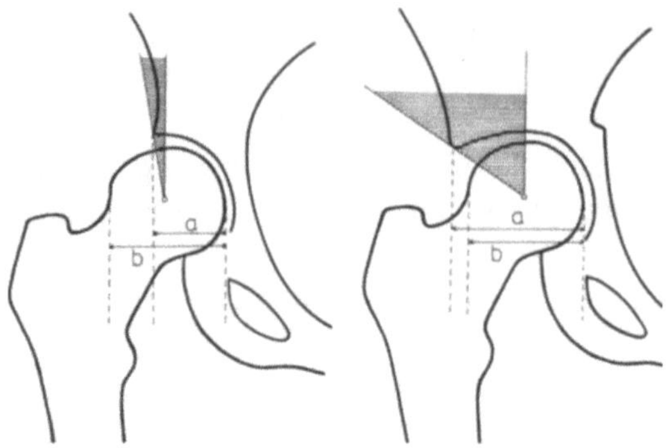

Fig. 2. Measurement of CE angle and acetabular roof covering the femoral head before (left) and after (right) osteotomy. (Femoral head coverage determined by the ratio of depth of the socket *a* to diameter of the femoral head *b*)

Change in the CE angle and the percentage of the acetabular roof covering the femoral head were determined roentgenologically (Fig. 2). In addition, the congruence of the joint, the width of the joint space, and bone structure, with particular attention to sclerosis due to weight-bearing, were evaluated. Although a standard AP picture does not show the covering of the femoral head in its full extent, the projection of the bone fragment edges permits a satisfactory assessment of the position of the acetabular roof. Measurement of the CE angle of Wiberg, which interprets mechanical width of the roof relative to the center of the head, was performed with the ischiometer of Müller. X-ray examination revealed a CE angle of more than 30° in 147 patients, 20°–30° in 11, and between 15° and 20° in 6 patients (Table 4). The results of pelvic osteotomy were still more impressive when the percentages of the acetabular roof coverage of the femoral head were compared pre- and postoperatively (Table 5). It was

Table 4. CE angle of the hip joint changed by osteotomy in 164 cases

Initial values	Results				
	up to 20°	21°–30°	31°–50°	above 50°	Totals
up to 0°	4	5	36	41	86
0°–5°	1	2	17	16	36
6°–10°	–	2	12	5	19
above 10°	1	2	9	11	23
Totals	6	11	74	73	164

Table 5. Change in femoral head coverage by osteotomy

		preoperative	postoperative	
Group I:	43	above 60%	85–99%:	5
			100% and more:	38
Group II:	65	50–60%	below 85%:	6
			85–99%:	11
			100% and more:	48
Group III:	43	below 50%	below 85%:	2
			85–99%:	8
			100% and more:	33
Group IV:	13	dislocations	below 85%:	1
			100% and more:	12

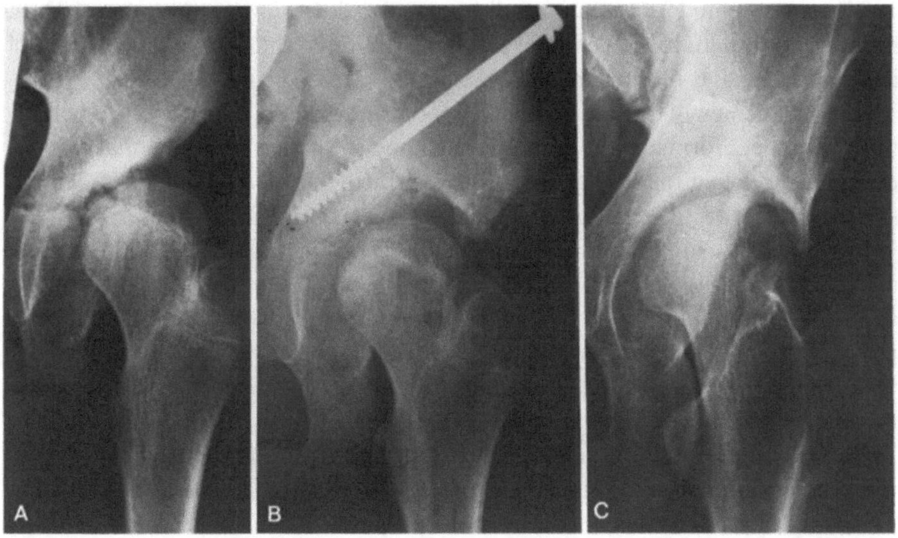

Fig. 3. (a) Dysplasia of the acetabulum of the left hip joint in a 12-year-old female. (b) Wide coverage of the femoral head following osteotomy. (c) Excellent adaptive remodeling of the newly formed roof, $3^1/_2$ years after pelvic osteotomy. Transposition of greater trochanter after osteotomy

Table 6

A) Change in the joint cartilage space

preoperative	postoperative	
small	small	–
25 pat.	medium	10
	large	15
medium	small	2
62 pat.	medium	15
	large	45
large	small	–
77 pat.	medium	6
	large	71

B) Change in the stress sclerosis of the acetabulum roof

preoperative	postoperative		
below $^1/_4$	below	$^1/_4$	1
79 pat.	below	$^1/_2$	4
	below	$^3/_4$	18
	full		56
below $^1/_2$	below	$^1/_4$	–
78 pat.	below	$^1/_2$	2
	below	$^3/_4$	16
	full		60
below $^3/_4$	below	$^1/_4$	–
7 pat.	below	$^1/_2$	–
	below	$^3/_4$	–
	full		7

100% or more in 131 cases, and did not fall below 80% in the others. Thus, normalization had been accomplished in all patients, since an 80% covering of the femoral head is found in healthy hip joints with a CE angle of 30°.

At first, the newly formed acetabular roof is not ideally congruent, but a bony roof, which conforms to the femoral head and is shaped by functional stresses due to remodeling of the flat osteotomy surface. Ideal remodeling, as demonstrated in Figure 3 observed after 43 months, occurred in 82% of cases.

In a dysplastic hip, pressure is not evenly distributed along the entire surface of the joint but is concentrated on small areas of contact between the femoral head and acetabulum. Thus it becomes unphysiologically high in relation to the unit area. Chiari's osteotomy assures distribution of pressure by providing a wide supporting surface and unloading the hip joint due to its biomechanical factors, especially the medial displacement. An increase in the joint cartilage space was noted radiologically in more than half of the patients at the time of reexamination (Table 6). Stress sclerosis of the head and acetabulum was impressively altered, as evidenced by more proportional loading, which was very small in almost all cases before operation. 94% of patients revealed marked widening of the stress sclerosis of the roof on follow-up examination. Moreover, bony irregularities and even occasional cysts observed preoperatively in the bone structure became normalized due to the improved stress conditions after osteotomy in almost all cases (Figs. 4 and 5).

In the clinical assessment of results hip joint mobility was compared before and after osteotomy (Table 7). Cases with a good femoral head contour (a) were separated from those with marked deformity of the femoral heads before

Table 7. Change in mobility after osteotomy, with the same classification of groupings as in Table 3. Preoperative mobility is evaluated as: good, moderate, poor. Postoperative mobility is evaluated as: increased, constant, decreased (+, =, −). Cases are divided between (a) good contour of femoral head, and (b) deformities of femoral head

	preoperative	postoperative (a) +	=	−	postoperative (b) +	=	−
Group I: (slight dysplasia)							
43 pat.	good		13	2		9	2
	moderate	2	4		5	2	1
	poor				3		
Group II: (moderate dysplasia)							
65 pat.	good		14	3		15	1
	moderate	5	2	1	7	8	3
	poor				5	1	
Group III: (severe dysplasia)							
43 pat.	good		7	1		7	2
	moderate	3			7	11	2
	poor	1			2		
Group IV: (dislocations)							
13 pat.	good		1	1		2	1
	moderate	1	2			5	

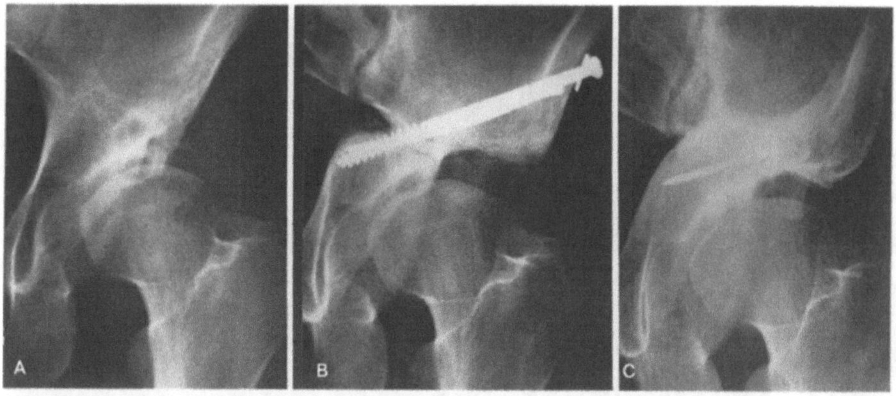

Fig. 4. (a) Severe dysplasia of the acetabulum of the left hip joint in a 19-year-old female. (b) Coverage of the femoral head in an osteotomy with very wide capsular interposition. (c) Remodeling of joint space with free mobility, 8 years after pelvic osteotomy

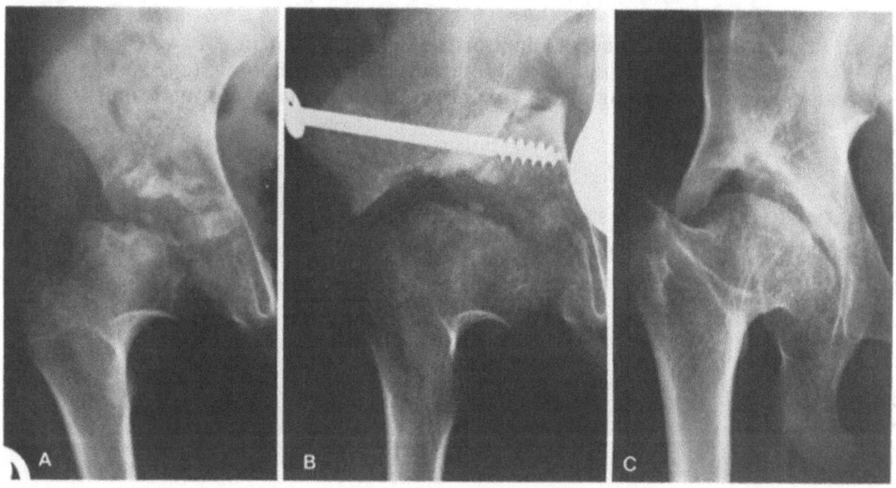

Fig. 5. (a) 6-year-old female. Severe dysplasia of the acetabulum of the right hip joint with deformed head, shortened femoral neck, and high riding greater trochanter following epiphyseal damage in early childhood. (b) Coverage of the femoral head with pelvic osteotomy. (c) Excellent adaptive remodeling of the newly formed roof, $6^1/_2$ years after osteotomy. The distal displacement osteotomy of the greater trochanter is indicated

operation (b). Table 7 shows that the great majority of patients had the same, or even some improvement in, movement, if preoperative movement was reasonably good. Poor preoperative movement was improved in nearly all cases. As can be seen in Table 7, of the 13 patients whose movement deteriorated postoperatively, 8 had slight limitation of their previously good abduction and 5 had limitation in all directions.

The pelvic osteotomy of Chiari has proved to be an efficient method in the treatment of dysplastic acetabula of children and juveniles. Particularly satisfying results are to be found if the contour of the femoral head is good and free mobility is present prior to osteotomy. But even under less favourable condi-

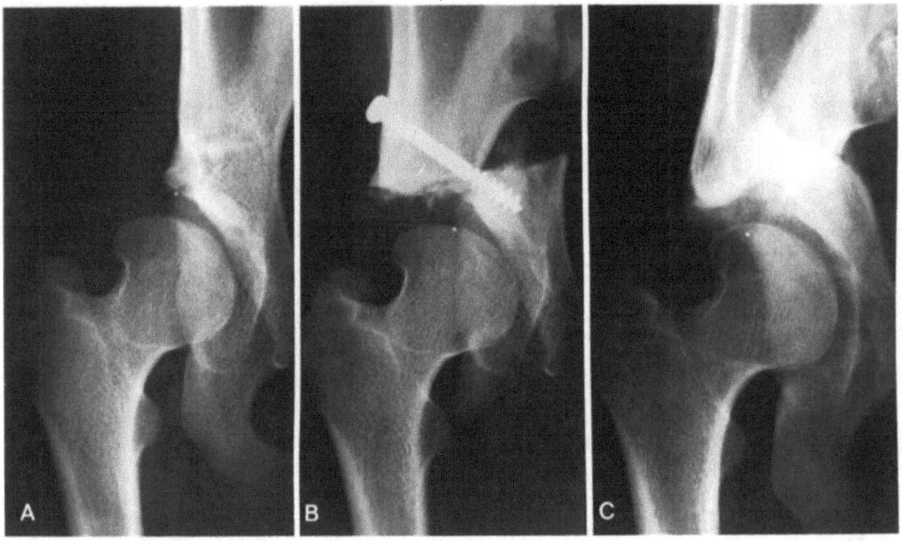

Fig. 6. (a) Dysplasia of the acetabulum of the right hip joint in a 14-year-old female. (b) Wide coverage of the femoral head following pelvic osteotomy. (c) Excellent adaptive remodeling and widening of the stress sclerosis of the newly formed roof, 10 years after osteotomy

tions, pelvic osteotomy results in good acetabular remodeling with satisfactory function of the joint. If the proper indications for the procedure are present it is not the method, but technical errors which produce failure.

Summary

Our experience with the Chiari osteotomy for correction of acetabular dysplasia in children and adolescents based on 164 operations has been reported. It is indicated in acetabular dysplasia with a CE angle of less than 10°. For rare cases with marked deformity of the femoral head, a CE angle between 10° and 20° is acceptable. Malposition of the proximal femur should be corrected as well. The effectiveness of the method is demonstrated by widening of the CE angle and improvement of the acetabular roof. Best results are achieved in cases with good contour of the femoral head and satisfactory movement preoperatively. Marked hip joint deformities are also substantially improved by the osteotomy. Early postoperative exercises made possible by stable internal fixation are very important. Flawless operative technique with proper selection of the osteotomy site and adequate displacement of fragments is essential for good results.

References

Chapchal, G.: Beckenosteotomie-Pfannendachplastik. Intern. Symp., January 30/31, 1965 Basel. Stuttgart: G. Thieme
Chiari, K.: Z. Orthop. **87,** 14 (1956)
Chiari, K.: Verh. Dtsch. Orthop. Ges. **47,** 504 (1960)
Chiari, K.: Verh. Dtsch. Ges. Orthop. u. Traumat. S. 193, 1970
Colton, C. L.: J. Bone Jt Surg. **54 B,** 4, 578 (1972)
Ebach, G.: Z. Orthop. **102,** 250 (1967)
Kollmann, K.: Z. Orthop. **102,** 262 (1967)
Müller, M. E.: Die hüftnahen Femurosteotomien. Stuttgart: G. Thieme 1971
Seyfarth, H.: Arch. orthop. UnfallChir. **61,** 1 (1967)
Strauß, H. J., Kreutzer, R., Daum, H.: Der Orthopäde **2,** 4 (1973)
Thomas, G.: Z. Orthop. **107,** 108 (1970)

Revised and updated English translation from the German edition *Der Orthopäde,* Vol. 2, pp. 245–249 (1973),

Experiences with Spherical Acetabular Osteotomy for the Correction of the Dysplastic Acetabulum

H. Wagner*

Dysplasia of the acetabulum consists of reduction of the depth of the acetabulum and shortening of its roof, a diminution of the superior and anterior articular surface, and also of a tilted position of the acetabulum. This leads to a reduction of that part of the articular surface which bears weight effectively. A thickening of the acetabular fossa develops during the growth period through insufficient centering of the forces of pressure acting on the dysplastic hip joint and can be detected quite frequently. It results in a lateralization of the pivoting point of the hip and thus elongates the lever arm of the body weight. The abnormal position of the proximal end of the femur in an increased valgus, and anteversion which generally occurs simultaneously, has a crucial and negative influence on pathologic stress conditions which occur in the hip joint due to the flattening and tilting of the dysplastic acetabulum. The characteristic malposition of the femoral neck shortens the effective lever arm of the pelvitrochanteric musculature and causes an eccentric orientation of the pressure forces in the hip joint. The shortening of the power arm increases the pressure in the joint, since the musculature of the shorter lever arm has to develop an increased tension in order to stabilize the hip joint while standing. The lateralization of the acetabular fossa with the elongated leverage of load increases in its turn the muscle tension necessary for the stabilization of the joint. This further increases the pressure in the joint.

Malformation and malposition of the acetabulum and the neck of the femur, by eccentric direction of the pressure, lead, therefore, to a transference of the pathologically increased pressure in the joint onto a pathologically diminished articular surface area. These stress conditions diminish the resistance of the joint and result in premature wear because the amount of pressure exceeds the mechanical firmness of the hyaline cartilage and damages its structure through overstress.

---

* Orthopädische Klinik des Wichernhauses Nuremberg/Altdorf (Head Physician: Prof. Dr. H. Wagner), Federal Republic of Germany

So far the problem of incongruence of the articular surfaces has not yet been taken into consideration. It is self-evident that a loss of congruence and a deformation of the femoral head and of the acetabulum, making the curvatures of the corresponding articular surfaces no longer identical, result in a reduction of the large area of gliding contact between the two elements of the joint. This incongruence reduces the portions of the articular surfaces which bear the pressure onto circumscribed areas in which the enormously increased pressure force wears out the articular cartilage. Thus the presence of a malposition of the acetabulum and of the femoral neck together with an incongruence of the articular surface create particularly unfavorable conditions for the durability of the hip joint. It must, however, be pointed out that, even if the articular surfaces of the femoral head and of the acetabulum are perfectly congruent, the mere shortening of the acetabular rim and the tilted position of the acetabulum can create serious pathologic stress conditions which will result in degenerative changes.

In a series of very impressive studies Pauwels has pointed out the importance of shortening the acetabular roof to create the faulty pressure distribution in the dysplastic acetabulum. If the femoral head is covered entirely, the vertical pressure force is distributed over the middle of the articular surface and thus the pressure force is small and evenly distributed over the joint (Fig. 1). With increased tilting of the acetabulum, its edge moves closer to the point where the pressure force has its main impact *(Druckstosspunkt,* "pressure-impact point") and the pressure force is transferred to a continually diminishing portion of the articular surface. The portion of the articular surface which bears the pressure can only be about 3 times as large as the distance of the pressure-impact point from the rim of the acetabulum. The pressure tension per surface area rises in proportion to the decrease of the pressure-bearing portion of the articular surface and, with a pathologically tilted acetabulum, attains values which exceed the resistance of the articular cartilage to friction.

In young patients the incomplete coverage of the femoral head caused by a dysplastic acetabulum can for a long time be functionally well compensated, especially if the congruence of the corresponding elements of the joint is

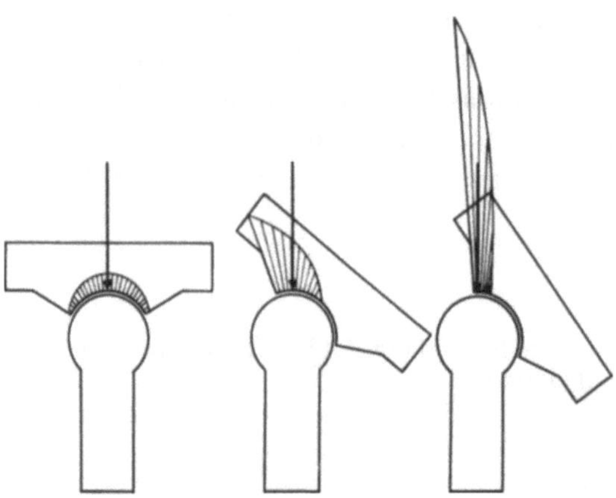

Fig. 1. Significance of a shortened acetabulum for the incorrect distribution of stress in the dysplastic hip joint (according to Pauwels). With increasing tilt of the acetabulum, the stress-bearing area of the articular surface diminishes and the pressure tensions per surface unit increase

unaltered. The shallow acetabulum with the coxa valga and anteversion allow free mobility of the hip joint, frequently even hypermobility. The efficient musculature of the young can compensate for these adverse leverage conditions and permit walking without limping or signs of fatigue. Finally, the great reserves of the articular cartilage in the young against friction prevents arthritic complaints even in cases of a diminished pressure-bearing surface. But these compensatory potentials are limited. Even with an originally excellent functional condition these pathologic stresses lead eventually to dysplastic arthrosis. After the cartilage reserves have been exhausted, arthritic complications set in, which in most cases increase rapidly. The reactive osseous changes with formation of cysts and osteophytic appositions cause a deformation of the joint elements, leading to incongruence and the faulty distribution of pressure, which accelerates decompensation of the joint (Fig. 2).

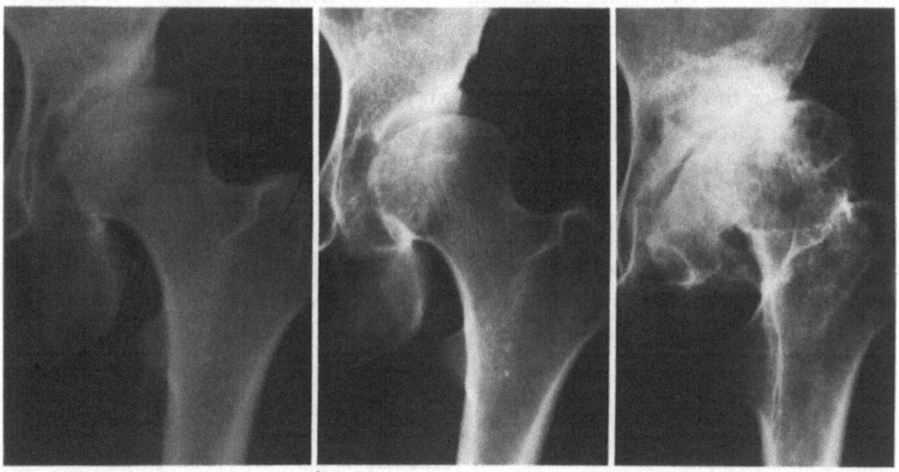

a b c

Fig. 2. Development of dysplastic arthrosis over a 20-year observation period. (a) A 22-year-old girl with normal clinical examination and no subjective symptoms. (b) At the age of 32, slight pain after long walks. (c) At the age of 45, a rapid increase in pain and difficulty in walking

The intertrochanteric derotation and adduction osteotomy can undoubtedly improve the faulty weight distribution in the dysplastic hip joint. By correcting the position of the neck of the femur, the power arm of the pelvitrochanteric musculature is elongated and thus the pressure in the joint diminishes. Simultaneously the direction of pull of the musculature changes with the removal of the greater trochanter from the pivotal point of the hip, thus transferring the resulting pressure force from the rim of the acetabulum medially and enlarging the pressure-bearing area of the articular surface. However, the possibilities for correction on the neck of the femur are very limited:

An intertrochanteric osteotomy can create ideal stress conditions within the hip joint only when the acetabular roof is sufficiently wide, with a CE angle of more than 20°. If the acetabulum is shallower, intertrochanteric osteotomy does not improve the stress conditions sufficiently. Due to the shortened acetabular roof the pressure-impact point of the resulting pressure force cannot, even by a vigorous correction of the position of the femoral neck, be transferred medially so far from the acetabular rim that an area of the articular surface large enough to bear pressure satisfactorily is obtained. Even an overcorrection of the position of the femoral neck has only a very slight effect on an additional change of direction of the resulting pressure force. It has the disadvantage that the high position of the greater trochanter decreases the tension and efficiency of the pelvitrochanteric musculature and that the cartilage rim of the femoral head, which is not very resistant to friction, is turned inward into the pressure zone. Overcorrections of the neck of the femur should, therefore, be avoided, since they do not improve, but rather reduce the durability of the hip joint as compared to a correction to the normal position.

Even if the head of the femur is ideally congruent, the shape of the proximal end of the femur in a dysplastic hip joint can be so distorted, mainly as a result of damage to the epiphysis in early childhood, that the ideal position of the femoral neck can no longer be determined with the CCD angle and the AT angle alone. In these cases the necessary correction can be determined from the positions of the articular surfaces and the greater trochanter.

In the normal anatomic condition the middle of the cranial articular surface of the femoral head is situated directly above the center of the joint or angled as much as 15° in the medial direction as measured on the a-p film when the neck of the femur is turned into the frontal plane. This central angle of the articular surface (CG angle) is a good orientation guide for assessing the position of the

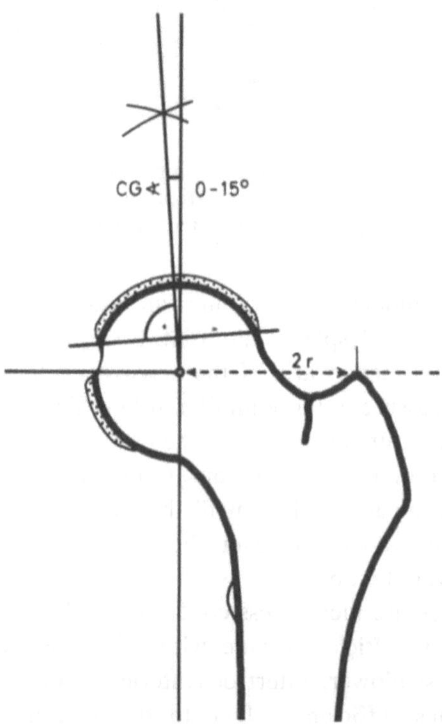

Fig. 3. Desired position of correction of the proximal end of the femur before acetabular osteotomy: the tip of the greater trochanter is level with the center of the femoral head and is turned in a lateral direction from it by 2–2.5 times the radius of the femoral head; the CG angle is 0–15°

articular surface of the femoral head and corresponds to the AC angle of the cranial articular surface of the acetabulum. The center of the cranial articular surface is situated on the femoral head in the middle, between the rim of the fovea of the head of the femur and the lateral border of the articular surface (Fig. 3).

If, for instance, after deformation of the femoral head in early childhood with damage to the epiphyseal growth centers, the epiphysis of the femoral head with the superior articular surface is rotated externally in a lateral direction, the fovea lies opposite to the superior articular surface of the acetabulum and the values of the CG angle become negative (Fig. 4). In this case an intertrochanteric adduction osteotomy is necessary to improve the congruence of the articular surfaces, independent of the position of the axis of the femoral neck and of the greater trochanter. The elevated position of the trochanter which can result from this can be corrected by a caudal displacement at the site of the trochanter.

In the case of a marked coxa valga, on the other hand, in which the epiphysis of the femoral head and the articular surface show a normal orientation, an intertrochanteric osteotomy is not advisable. The lowering of the neck of the femur would turn the rim of the articular surface of the femoral head into the

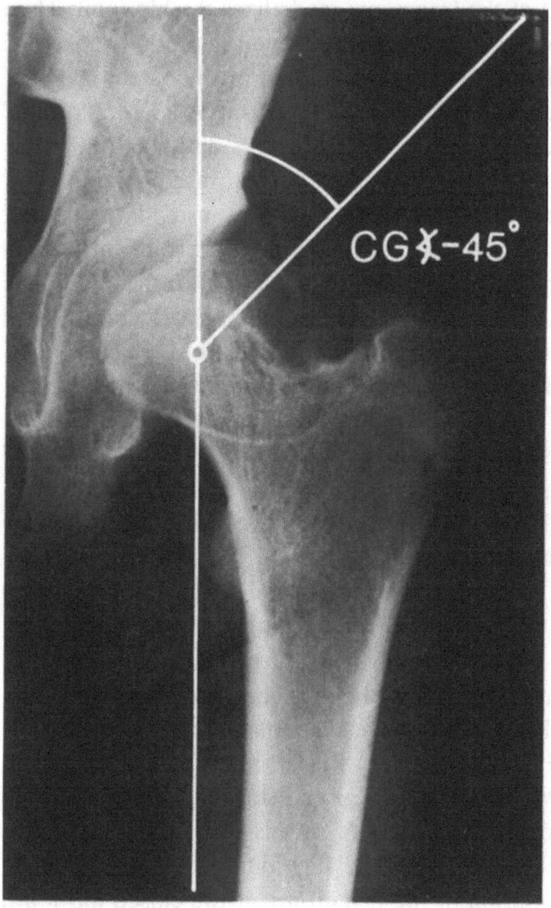

Fig. 4. Lateral twist of the epiphysis of the femoral head with a negative CG angle after damage to the epiphysis in early childhood

pressure zone and thus change the congruence in the articular space for the worse. In such a case the functional effects of the coxa valga should, therefore, be corrected by a displacement of the greater trochanter.

The ideal position of the neck of the femur, which one should try to obtain before correcting the dysplastic acetabulum, is defined as follows:

1. The CG angle of the femoral head should be 0–15°
2. The tip of the greater trochanter should be level with the center of the femoral head and its position should be lateral to the center of the head by 2–2.5 times the radius of the femoral head.
3. The anteversion angle of the femur should be 10–15°.

If, after a correction of the proximal end of the femur, the femoral head is still imcompletely covered, with a CE angle of less than 20°, optimal reconstruction is only possible by enlarging the acetabular roof.

For the correction of a dysplastic acetabulum in juveniles and young adults, where classic "plastic operations" of the roof of the acetabulum and Salter's innominate osteotomy are no longer advisable, Chiari's pelvic osteotomy has proved to be a dependable method, which, even in cases of serious dysplasias, still allows complete coverage of the femoral head. A further advantage of this method is that the displacement of the fragments medializes the hip joint. Thus it moves closer to the center of gravity of the body, even if the medialization does not correspond to the full extent of the dislocation of the osteotomy surfaces, as more than half of this displacement is brought about by a lateral turn of the proximal fragment with a gap of the sacroiliac suture. A disadvantage of the pelvic osteotomy is that between the proximal osteotomy surface containing the roof and the femoral head, the superior joint capsule, instead of hyaline articular cartilage, serves as an interpositum and corresponding joint surface for the femoral head and thus enters the main pressure zone of the hip joint. Furthermore, the turning of the distal fragment in the medial direction causes the dysplastic acetabulum, which is already strongly slanted but which is lined with hyaline cartilage, to become even steeper and to be even further exempt from stress. This constitutes a loss of function because in a young patient the articular cartilage is still very resistant to friction.

If both the femoral head and the acetabulum are congruent, and if the hyaline articular surface of the acetabulum is sufficiently large, these disadvantages can be avoided through acetabular osteotomy (Fig. 5).

In this method the dysplastic acetabulum, in the form of a cartilaginous-osseous, hemispheric bowl, is cut out of the pelvic isthmus, down to the obturator foramen while the joint capsule is unopened, and is then turned or folded outwards in the anterolateral direction until the femoral head is completely covered. The osteotomy is performed with the help of a special spoon-shaped chisel (manufactured by Robert Mathys, CH-2544 Bettlach) with a spherical surface which, when penetrating into the pelvic isthmus on a global surface, cuts around the acetabulum parallel to the articular space. Sets of chisels with different radii of curvature are available for varying radii of the hip joint. A roentgen-image intensifier is necessary for orientation of the osteotomy at the closed hip joint.

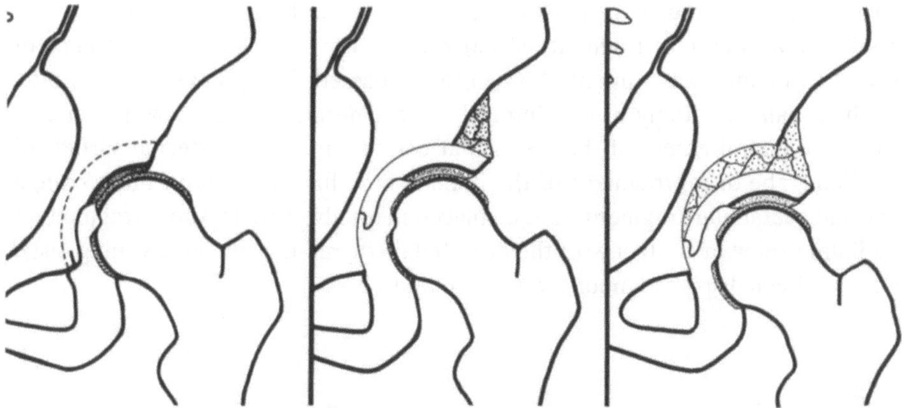

Fig. 5. Schematic representation of acetabular osteotomy types I and II: (a) A cut around the dysplastic acetabulum is performed on a spherical osteotomy surface, and the isolated acetabulum (b) (type I) is pulled over the femoral head in the form of a spherical bowl or (c) (type II) is folded out and over the femoral head with a slight elongating effect. The osteotomy gap is filled with autologous cancellous bone grafts

The thickness of the bone layer remaining on the acetabulum must be at least 10 mm to avoid a fracture of the acetabular bowl reliably. Over the years experience has shown that, even if the layer is 15 mm thick, a nutritional deficiency of the isolated acetabular cavity does not occur.

After the osteotomy has been accomplished, two pairs of spreaders are inserted into the space created by the osteotomy and the acetabulum is slowly loosened and pulled over the femoral head. If no major gap is created in the space resulting from the osteotomy by pulling out the acetabulum, the pivoting point of the hip joint remains unchanged. When the acetabulum is unfolded, it is also displaced in a distal direction by which means it can be lengthened by as much as 2 cm. Depending on the circumstances, either one or the other dislocation modus may be preferred. For assessment of a sufficient coverage of the femoral head during the dislocation of the acetabulum, a Kirschner wire is inserted into the osteotomy space parallel to the connecting line between the two anterior superior iliac spines, which greatly facilitates evaluation on the image intensifier.

The acetabulum is then fixed in the desired corrected position by means of two hook plates which are screwed tightly on the outside of the upper part of the ilium. The gaping osteotomy space and the protruding edge of the acetabular cavity are filled with corticocancellous bone chips from the iliac crest.

Osteosynthesis makes it possible to begin movement immediately after the operation. After 2–3 days partial weight-bearing of 15 kg on the leg can be practised on a scale. Loading the leg with half the body weight is usually permitted after 8 weeks, and with full body weight after 4 months.

The configuration of the hemipelvis may be such that the mechanics of the joint could be improved by displacing the center of hip motion medially. This can be achieved by combining the acetabular osteotomy with a medial displacement osteotomy through the isthmus of the ilium.

After the previously described acetabular osteotomy is completed, the mobilized acetabular fragment is separated from the ilium by a fragment spreader or similar instrument. A Gigli saw is passed through the greater sciatic notch and an osteotomy of the ilium, the saw emerging at or a few millimeters above the lateral extent of the acetabular osteotomy on the external surface of the ilium. The distal fragment of the ilium is mobilized from both the proximal iliac and acetabular fragments and displaced medially. The proximal fragment of the ilium is now in contact with the acetabular fragment as the intervening distal ilium has been displaced medially. (Figs. 6 and 12–14).

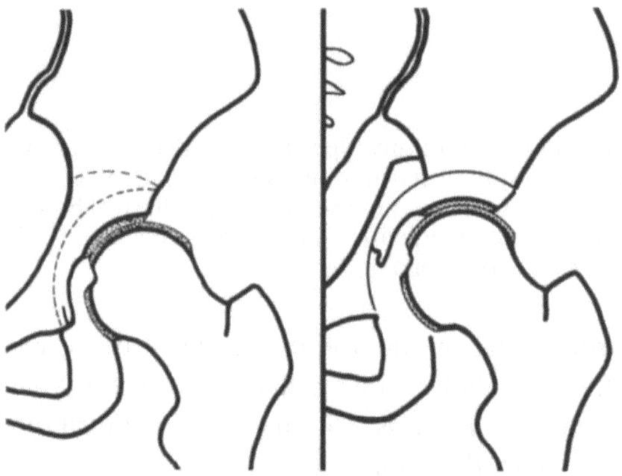

Fig. 6. Acetabular osteotomy type III: The spherical osteotomy cut around the dysplastic acetabulum is combined with a transverse osteotomy of the isthmus ilei, by which means after redirection of the acetabulum the hip joint can be shifted medially, closer to the center of gravity

The acetabular fragment is rotated laterally and anteriorly so that it protrudes from the proximal iliac fragment. After the three fragments are correctly orientated so that they improve the CE angle and medialize the hip joint, the acetabular fragment is fixed to the proximal ilium. Two 2.5-mm-diameter Kirschner wires are fixed into place between the crest of the ilium and the superior cut surface of the acetabular fragment, taking care that these do not protrude through the acetabular fragment into the hip joint. The two Kirschner wires, which are 2–3 cm apart, are joined by a small contoured semitubular plate with both ends curved to grasp the Kirschner wires. A single 4.5-mm cortical screw is used to fix the plate to the ilium. When the plate compresses the Kirschner wires against the ilium, the medially displaced acetabular fragment is locked into place. Small gaps among the three fragments are filled with cancellous bone grafts. Adequate stability is achieved so that early motion may be permitted.

An incontestable advantage of acetabular osteotomy is the fact that the hyaline cartilaginous articular surface of the dysplastic acetabulum is brought from a pathologically tilted position with unphysiologic stress conditions into the normal position with complete covering of the femoral head. Conditions are thus created which approximate the normal anatomic condition and which, according to our experience with prearthritic deformities, counteract most reliably the development of symptoms of wear (Hackenbroch).

The disadvantage of this method lies in the fact that the operation is technically more complicated than the innominate osteotomy and that a good curvature of the joint elements with a sufficiently large acetabulum are a prerequisite. Acetabular osteotomy cannot be performed on acetabular dysplasias with only rudimentary remnants of the original articular surfaces because they cannot adequately cover the femoral head in the normal position with a sufficiently large hyaline cartilage articular surface. Furthermore, for the purpose of adjustment to normal conditions, acetabular osteotomy is not suitable for correcting cases where the curvatures of the elements of the joint are seriously deformed. The deformation of the articular surface will persist. The appropriate treatment for such cases is pelvic osteotomy, which, even in very advanced conditions, does not aim at morphologic correction, but rather at functional adjustment without altering the anatomic deformity.

The decision to operate, too, is more difficult for acetabular osteotomy, at least psychologically. Its best prognosis is in joints which cause few complaints and which have little wear, a state in which pain and functional disorder do not play an important role in indicating surgery. In comparison, pelvic osteotomy possesses a wide spectrum of indications, even in cases of pronounced arthritic changes with painful functional disorder.

Acetabular osteotomy and pelvic osteotomy, therefore, are not methods which compete, but rather which complement each other. Each has its clearly defined indications.

The experiences with acetabular osteotomy for the correction of the dysplastic acetabulum reported here are based on reexaminations of a consecutive series of 88 hip joints in 76 patients, who were operated on between 1966 and 1976. Fortunately, all could be reexamined. In evaluating our material (Table 1), the

Table 1. Analysis of the patients

ACETABULAR OSTEOTOMIES 1966 - 1976

88 HIP JOINTS IN 76 PATIENTS
(12 BILATERAL)

71 FEMALE
5 MALE

CONCOMITANT SURGERY:

INTERTROCHANTERIC OSTEOTOMIES	32
INTERTROCH. DOUBLE-OSTEOTOMIES	7
DISPLACEMENT OF MAJOR TROCHANTER	29

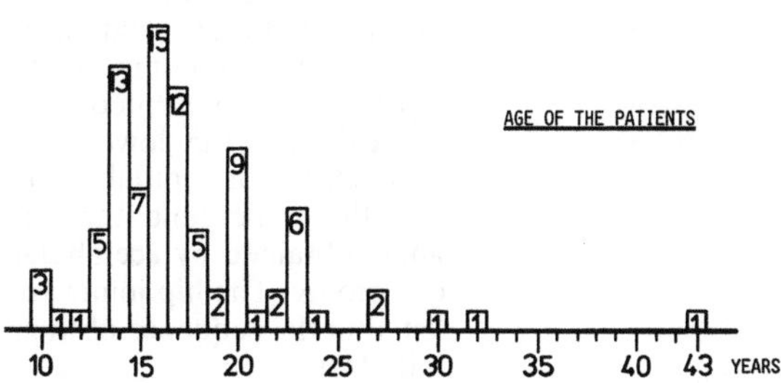

high percentage of female patients with a ratio of 14,2:1 is noteworthy. Acetabular osteotomy was performed 64 times unilaterally and 12 times bilaterally in separate sessions. In 32 cases intertrochanteric osteotomy with adduction "varisation" and derotation or "valgisation" of the proximal end of the femur were necessary prior to acetabular osteotomy. In 29 cases a trochanteric displacement osteotomy, either carried out alone or else in conjunction with intertrochanteric osteotomy, was necessary. In 7 cases an intertrochanteric double-osteotomy (Wagner) was performed.

The age of the great majority of patients at the time of operation was between 13 and 20 years, i.e., at a stage of development when the Y-line is already closed, but the hip joint still free of arthritic changes. Acetabular osteotomy was performed on 5 patients aged 25 or more, since in these cases the articular surfaces were freely mobile and ideally congruent and no arthritic reaction had as yet set in, so that a far-reaching normalization as a result of the operation could be expected. The best age for acetabular osteotomy, according to our experience, is between 14 and 18 years. At this age it is possible to determine with certainty the magnitude of the dysplasia, including its significance for dysplastic arthrosis. In addition, the generally free mobility of the joint without any symptoms of deterioration vouchsafes a good prognosis.

In all 88 hip joints, the CE angle (Table 2) before operation was less than 20°; in 71 hip joints it was less than 10° and in 25 hip joints it was less than 0°. Almost all acetabular osteotomies greatly improved or even normalized the CE angle; only in 3 hip joints was the CE angle after surgery still less than 20°, in spite of considerable improvement (Table 2).

After acetabular osteotomy the mobility of the hip joints was generally very good, especially when compared to their initial condition. The great majority of joints were freely mobile or hypermobile; the hinge mobility of only two joints was below 90°. Mobility after acetabular osteotomy does not depend on the original amount of the dysplasia nor on the extent of the surgical acetabular correction. Mobility depends rather on the extent of movement before the intervention and whether the postoperative range of motion exercises are carried out regularly. The effect of acetabular osteotomy with regard to function and durability of the joint (Figs. 7–14) can be judged from the free mobility of the

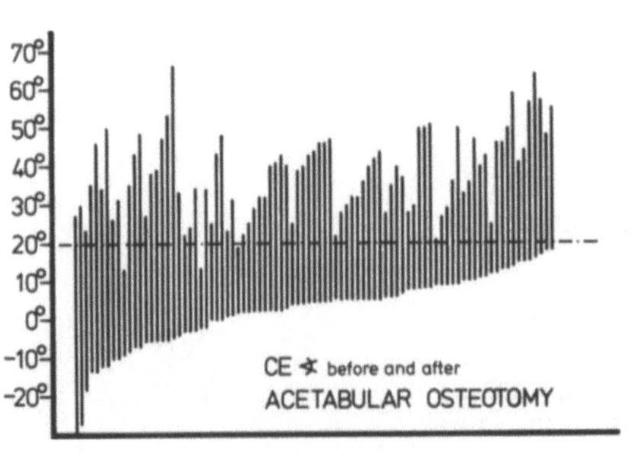

Table 2. Graphic representation of the CE angles of 88 hip joints before and after acetabular osteotomy. Each hip joint is represented by a vertical line, the lower end designating the initial angle and the upper end the CE angle obtained by acetabular osteotomy. The hip joints are listed in the sequence of their initial CE angle

hip joint and the considerable correction of the CE angle and the covering of the femoral head with a true articular surface.

Complications: Fortunately, in the present series of 88 hip joints, not one serious complication during surgery occurred. In one case a wound hematoma in an 18-year-old female patient had to be treated on the 5th day after operation. Continuous bleeding required reopening of the wound on the 13th and 32nd days postoperatively. She healed with an ideal roentgenogram and free mobility of the joint. After initial treatment of the hematoma this patient received antibiotic therapy. All other incisions healed without complications; no antibiotic prophylaxis was carried out.

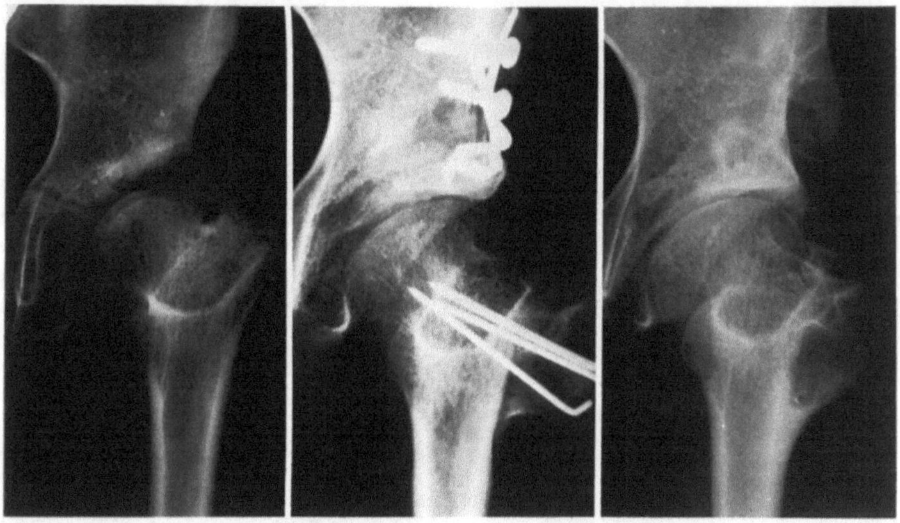

a b c

Fig. 7. Acetabular osteotomy type I in a 14-years-old girl: (b) 8 weeks and (c) 4 years after acetabular osteotomy and displacement osteotomy of the greater trochanter

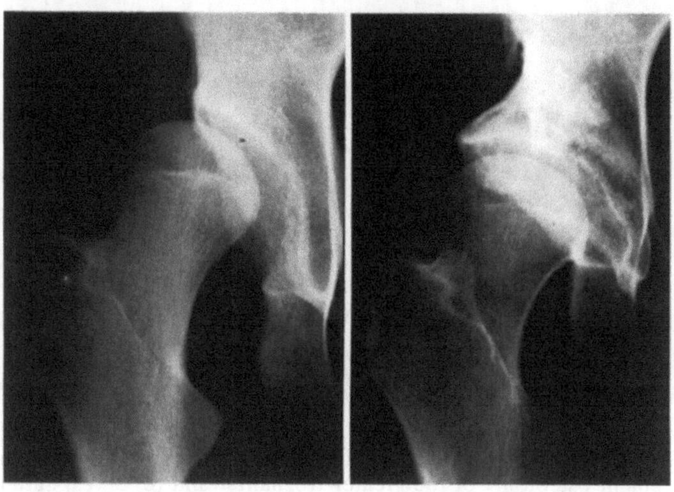

Fig. 8. Acetabular osteotomy type I in a 14-year-old girl 8 years after surgery

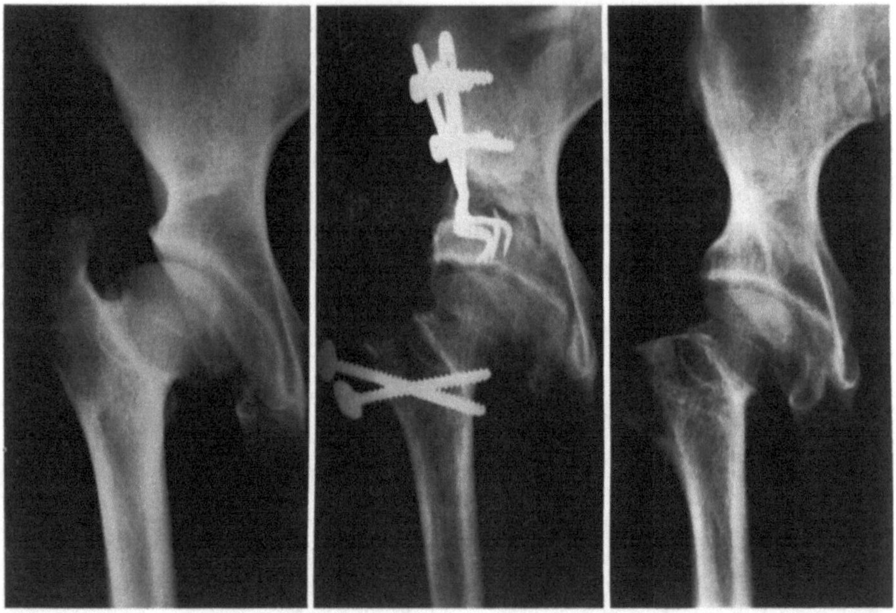

a b c

Fig. 9. Acetabular osteotomy type II in a 16-year-old girl (b) 8 weeks and (c) 4 years after acetabular osteotomy and displacement osteotomy of the greater trochanter

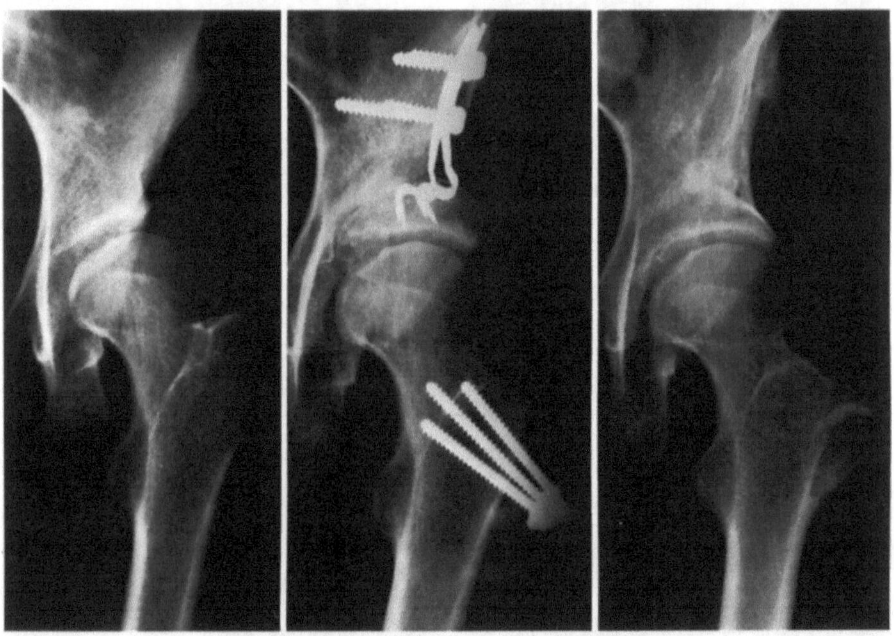

a b c

Fig. 10. Acetabular osteotomy type II in a 13-year-old girl (b) 8 weeks after acetabular osteotomy and displacement osteotomy of the greater trochanter and (c) 5 years after surgery

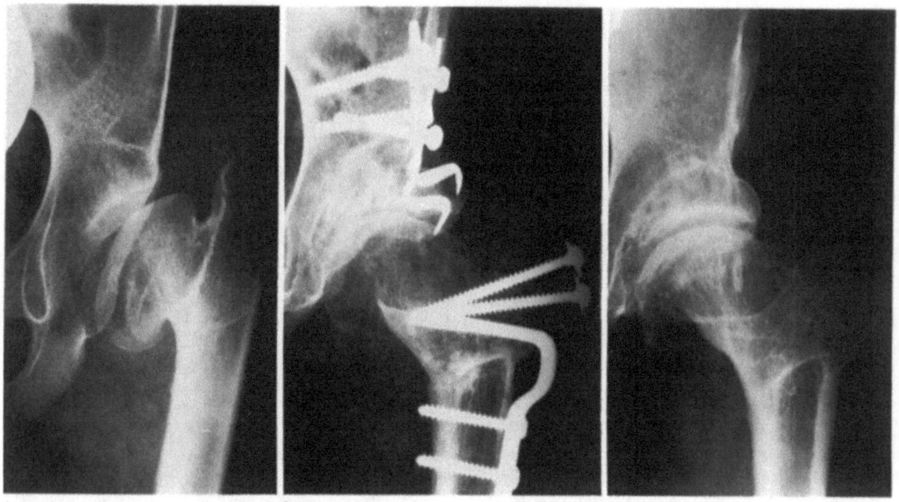

Fig. 11. Borderline indication for acetabular osteotomy type II in a 15-year-old girl (b) 8 weeks after acetabular osteotomy and intertrochanteric double osteotomy and (c) 5 years after surgery

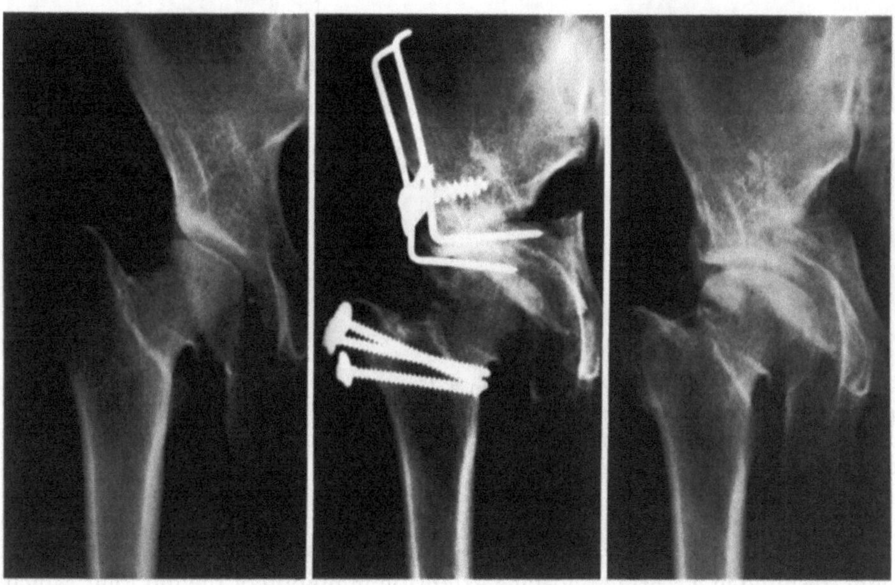

Fig. 12. Acetabular osteotomy type III in a 23-year-old female (b) 8 weeks after acetabular osteotomy and displacement osteotomy of the greater trochanter and (c) 2 years after surgery

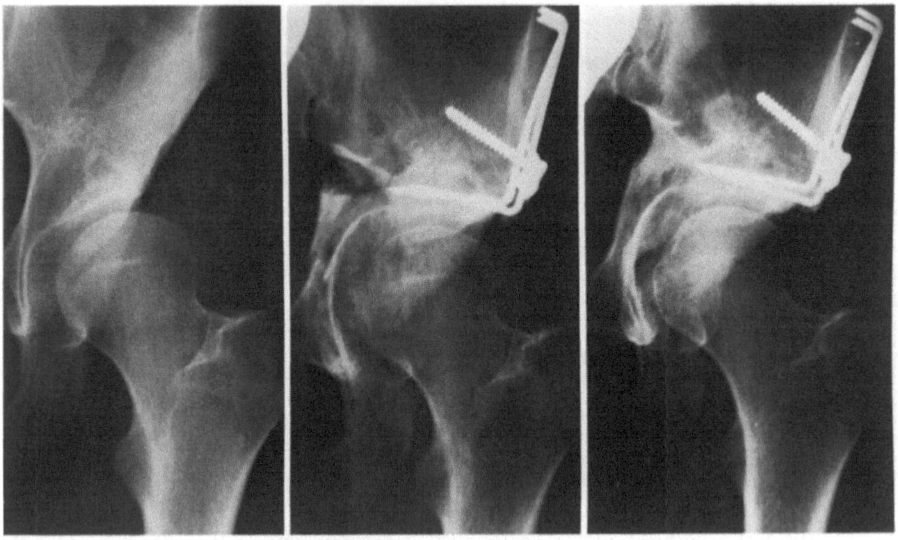

a b c

Fig. 13. Acetabular osteotomy type III in a 17-year-old girl (b) 8 weeks after surgery and (c) 2 years after surgery

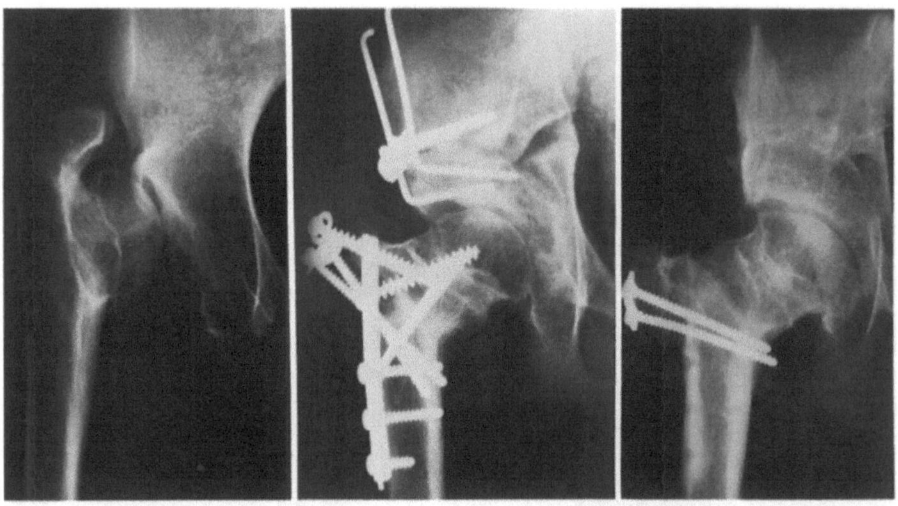

a b c

Fig. 14. Acetabular osteotomy type III in a 13-year-old girl (b) 5 months after intertrochanteric double osteotomy and 8 weeks after acetabular osteotomy; (c) 18 months after acetabular osteotomy and 3 months after additional displacement osteotomy of the greater trochanter

In four other patients the healing process, with unsatisfactory results in movement, resulted in a scarred endstage extension inhibition of the hip joint, which could be corrected by reopening the scar when the metal was removed. In two cases we also resected periarticular ossifications which affected mobility while the fixation devices were removed.

In an earlier series of operations when the present instrumentarium was not available and not osteosynthesis but immobilization in plaster was carried out, we observed a fracture of an overly thin acetabular bowl in two patients. This complication has not occurred since we keep the thickness of the layer of bone remaining around the acetabulum to a minimum of 10 mm. A nutritional deficiency of the larger shell of bone has never been observed.

Summary

The principle, indications, and technique of spherical acetabular osteotomy for the correction of the dysplastic acetabulum are described. Experience with a series of operations on 88 hip joints is reported:

Acetabular spherical osteotomy is indicated and has proved successful for the correction of the dysplastic acetabulum in cases without marked loss of congruence in the joint elements. A prerequisite for the operation is a sufficiently large cartilage articular surface in the acetabulum with which the femoral head can be covered in the normal position. This method creates conditions in the hip joint which resemble its normal state. Therefore, one can expect a decisive positive influence on the durability of the hip joint over a long period of time.

References

Chiari, K.: Verh. Dtsch. Orthop. Ges. **84,** 254 (1953)
Chiari, K.: Z. Orthop. **87,** 14 (1956)
Chiari, K.: Verh. Dtsch. Ges. Orthop. u. Traumat. **56,** 193 (1969)
Hackenbroch, M.: Die Arthrosis deformans der Hüfte. Grundlagen und Behandlung. S. 144, Leipzig: Thieme
Hackenbroch, M.: Verh. Dtsch. Orthop. Ges. **88,** 28 (1957)
Hackenbroch, M.: In: Chapchal, G.: Beckenosteotomie – Pfannendachplastik. Stuttgart: Thieme 1965
Pauwels, F.: Z. Orthop. **79,** 305 (1950)
Wagner, H.: In: Chapchal, G.: Beckenosteotomie – Pfannendachplastik. Stuttgart: Thieme 1965
Wagner, H.: In: The Hip. S. 45–66, St. Louis: Mosby 1976
Wagner, H.: Orthopäde **6,** 145 (1977)

Revised and updated English translation from the German edition *Der Orthopäde,* Vol. 2, pp. 253–259 (1973), © Springer-Verlag 1973

Comparison of Pelvic Osteotomies in the Treatment of Congenital Hip Dislocation

D. C. Stephens* and G. D. MacEwen**

In the child beyond walking age, several types of pelvic osteotomy have been popularized in order to improve the mechanics of the hip joint and to retard the development of osteoarthritis. Each procedure has its own rationale and method, and accordingly, the indications vary somewhat for each type of procedure. Our purpose is to review the principles of patient assessment and to discuss the Pemberton pericapsular osteotomy, the Steel triple innominate osteotomy, Sutherland's osteotomy and the shelf acetabuloplasty.

Although each of the procedures discussed is an extraarticular osteotomy, the capacity of hip stiffness remains and the patient's preoperative hip motion must be optimum. Contractures present about the hip must be taken into account and in cases where the femoral head is proximally displaced, preoperative traction may be necessary in order to avoid placing excessive pressure on the femoral head and inducing avascular necrosis.

The AP pelvis X-ray is the major determinant in choosing the procedure which best solves a particular problem. The acetabular index and CE angle are important in assessing femoral-acetabular relationships. One must also assess the amount of anteversion and the state of femoral head vascularity and determine whether the acetabulum or femoral head, or both, is more deficient. A standing AP pelvis X-ray demonstrates femoral-acetabular relationships under weight-bearing conditions and also points out any limb length discrepancy which may be present. In addition AP pelvis X-rays with varying amounts of hip abduction demonstrate the degree to which a hip will center. Each of the procedures discussed below requires that the hip center on abduction.

Pemberton Osteotomy

With the Pemberton osteotomy, the acetabular roof is changed in direction and shape by performing a pericapsular iliac osteotomy hinged on the triradiate

* Associate Surgeon, A. I. duPont Institute, Wilmington, Delaware, USA
** Medical Director and Surgeon-in-Chief, A. I. duPont Institute, Wilmington, Delaware, USA

cartilage. The change in direction of the acetabular roof is thus much greater than in the innominate procedure of Salter where the lateral rotation of the roof of the acetabulum is at the symphysis pubis. It is indicated with moderate to moderately severe acetabular dysplasia where there is a major true deficiency in the angle of the cartilagenous roof. The dysplastic hip with enlarged acetabular volume is ideal for this procedure.

Fig. 1 shows the X-ray of a patient well suited for the Pemberton osteotomy once reduction has been accomplished. The deformity should be confirmed by arthrogram because the true cartilage model may be intact and would therefore be grossly distorted by the procedure.

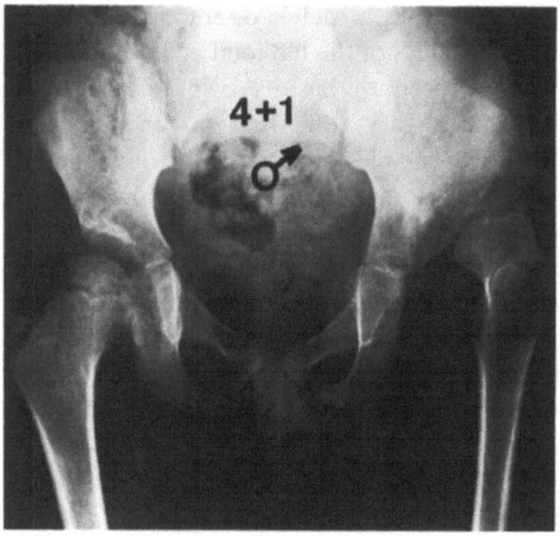

Fig. 1. This 4-year-old male has had no previous treatment. Note the enlarged dysplastic acetabulum; once reduction is accomplished, a Pemberton osteotomy will improve hip stability

The Pemberton osteotomy requires a more extensive surgical exposure and is technically more difficult than the Salter procedure. The level of the cut is important and must be carried posteriorly into the triradiate cartilage. By altering the depth of the osteotomy on the inside as compared to the outside cortex of pelvis, one can direct the distal fragment either more anteriorly or laterally as needed. It is essential that the cut not enter the acetabulum and injure the acetabular cartilage. The pre- and postoperative X-rays of a patient are seen in Figs. 2 and 3. Because the acetabular roof is changed with this procedure, there is potential for hip stiffness following surgery. Consequently, as full a range of motion as possible should precede the operation, and postoperative immobilization should not exceed 6 weeks. Since the acetabular volume is decreased with this procedure, there is considerable risk of increasing acetabular pressure on the femoral head. The procedure should therefore be preceded by femoral traction until the head is level with the final desired position.

The incongruity produced in the acetabulum should correct with remodeling in the growing child, but this procedure may produce a stiff hip in the older child in whom the acetabular incongruity is aggravated and limited capacity for

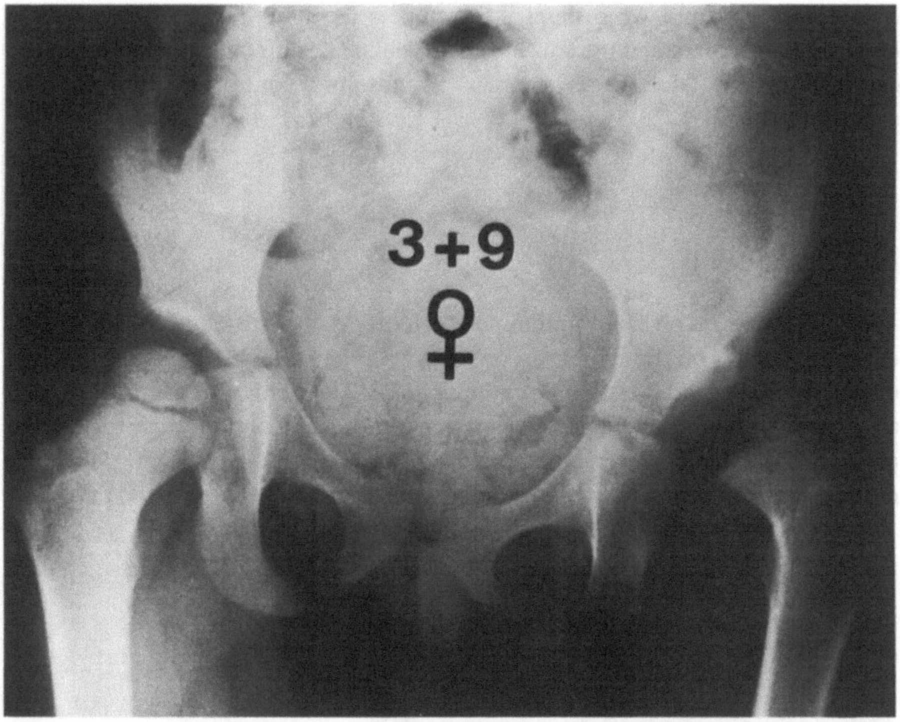

Fig. 2. A 3 year, 9 month old female prior to Pemberton pericapsular osteotomy

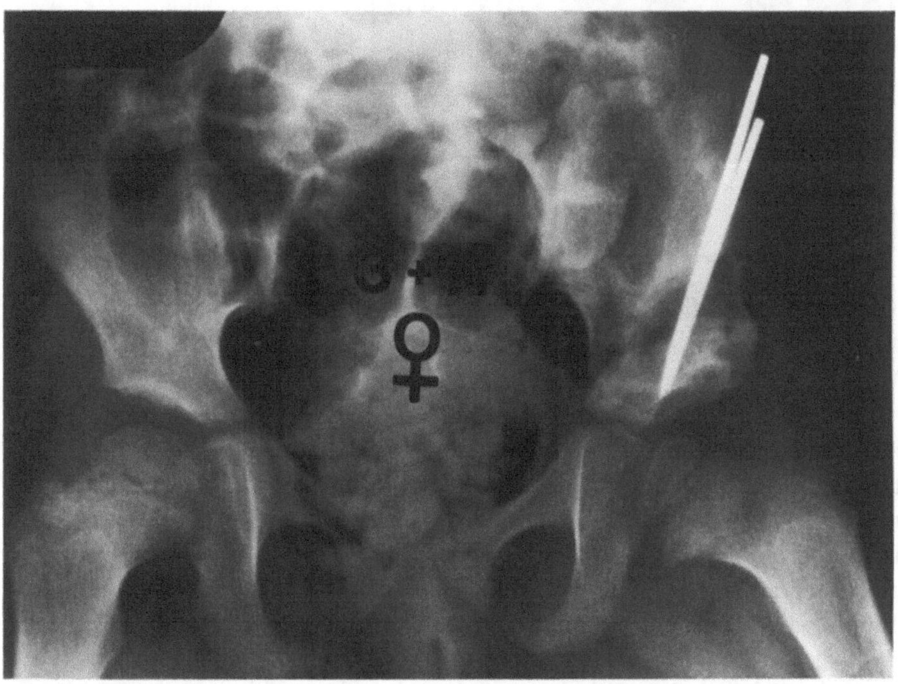

Fig. 3. Patient seen in Fig. 2 following Pemberton osteotomy and pin fixation of the inferior fragment

remodeling remains. Accordingly, the upper age limit for the procedure is between 8–10 years and the lower limit 2 years. Closure of the triradiate in the cartilage in the adolescent becomes an absolute contraindication for this procedure.

Steel Osteotomy

This procedure involves an innominate osteotomy, but instead of a single iliac cut which rotates on the symphysis pubis as with the Salter procedure, additional osteotomies are made through both pubic rami. The ischial cut is made through an incision in the buttock and the superior ramus is divided through the medial aspect of the Smith-Petersen approach. These osteotomies then allow free motion and redirection of the acetabular segment to allow better head coverage. The osteotomy is depicted in the model in Fig. 4.

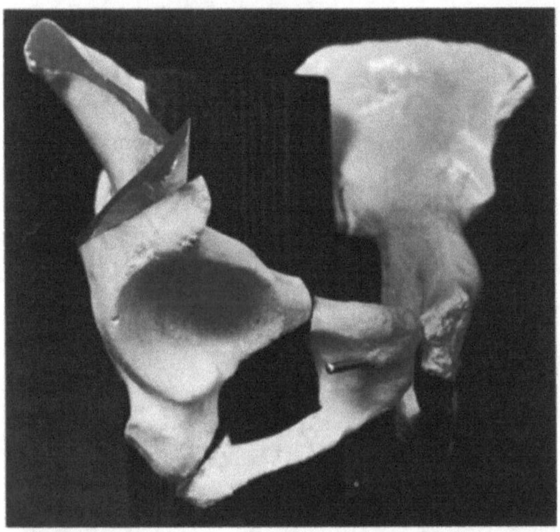

Fig. 4. Steel triple innominate osteotomy. Cuts are at a distance from acetabulum

This procedure is indicated in the older child with a markedly dysplastic acetabulum in whom a concentric reduction can be accomplished. It should not be done if the problem can be corrected with a simpler procedure. The preoperative X-ray of a 12 year, 9 month old female who underwent this procedure is seen in Fig. 5. The postoperative appearance with pin fixation incorporating the iliac graft is seen in Fig. 6. An advantage of the procedure is that the osteotomies are carried out at some distance from the hip joint and the articular cartilage surface is preserved after being redirected. Patients with CDH as a group have done better with the procedure than those with a paralytic or neuromuscular disease in whom an underlying reason favoring redislocation persists.

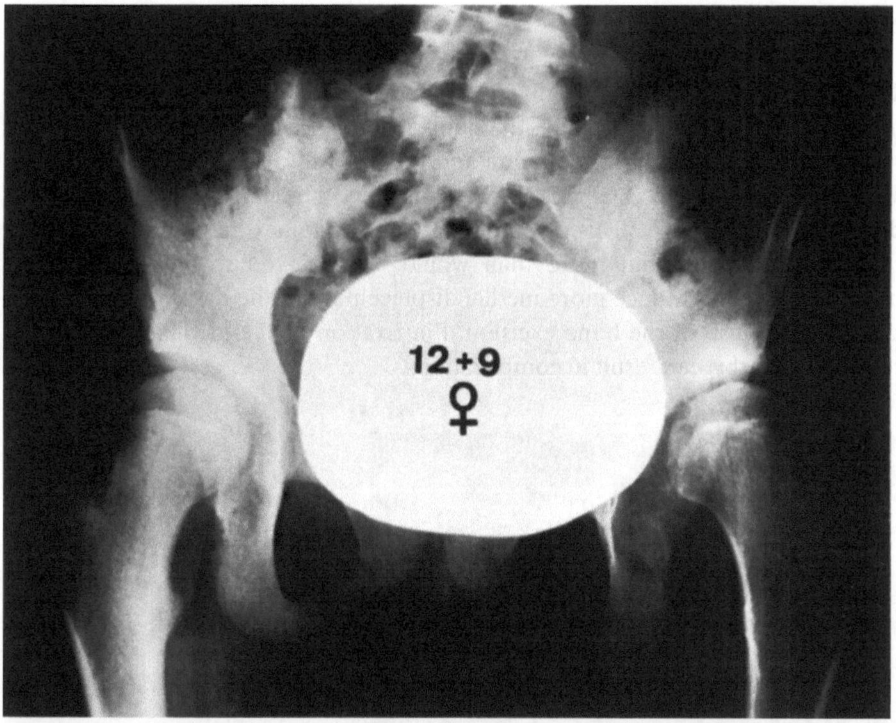

Fig. 5. A 12 year, 9 month old female prior to triple innominate osteotomy

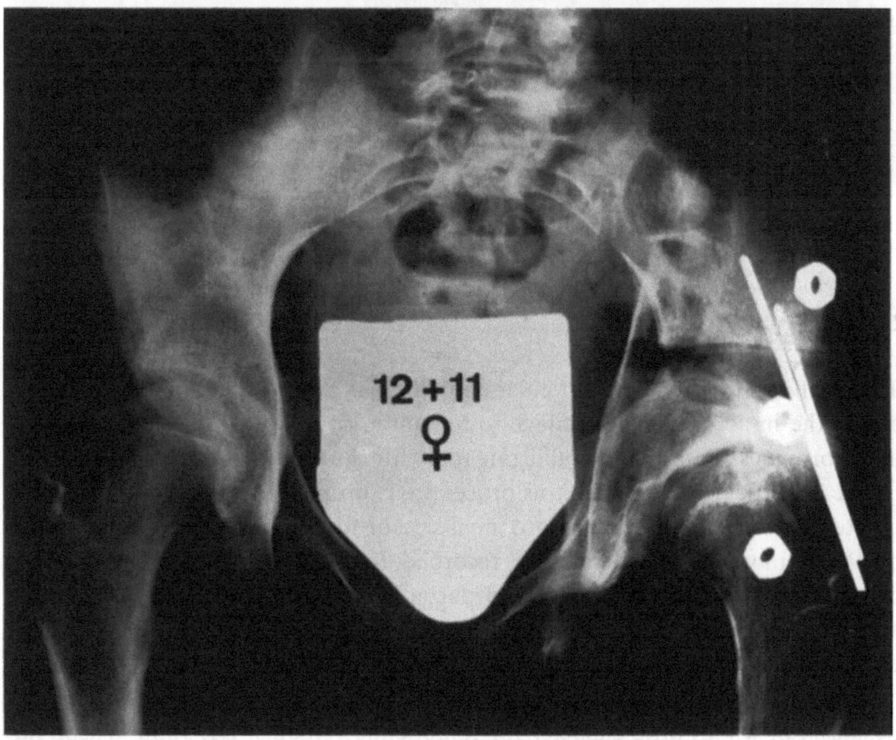

Fig. 6. Postoperative X-ray demonstrates improved head coverage

Sutherland Osteotomy

This procedure is similar in principle and indication to the Steel osteotomy; however, the osteotomy through the pubis is made from above. The cut passes just medial to the obturator foramen and just lateral to the symphysis pubis. A section of bone up to 2 cm is removed to allow medical displacement of the distal fragment (Fig. 7). This osteotomy allows for somewhat less rotation than the Steel procedure but more than would be achieved with an innominate procedure. It can produce more medial displacement of the distal fragment than the Steel because of the bone excision. Pin fixation of the medial osteotomy is required, and this can result in complications.

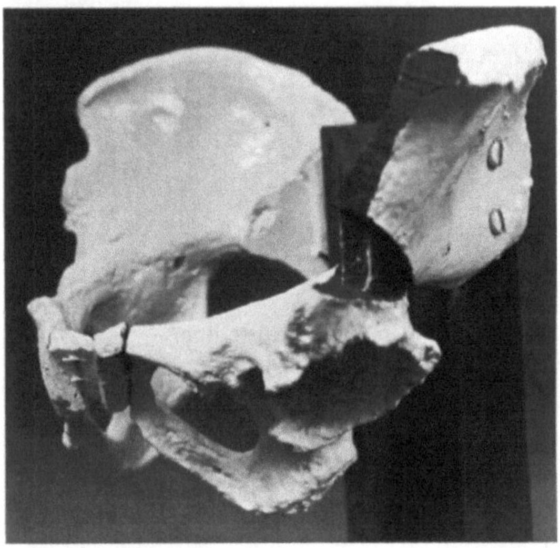

Fig. 7. Sutherland innominate osteotomy. Medial pubic osteotomy requires pin fixation

Shelf Procedure

The shelf was the first extraarticular containment procedure to be developed. It allows the intact articular cartilage to remain in contact with the femoral head, and it provides a buttress or stabilizing force for the femoral head.

The principal problem with this procedure is proper placement of the shelf. It is often placed too high on the proximal side of the pelvis so that it fails to support the femoral head and in time is resorbed. In order to be placed properly, the capsule must be stripped down and partially excised in order to localize the acetabulum level accurately. At that point one can pry down the outer pelvic cortex and buttress it with extra bone.

This procedure is most useful in the older child 10–18 years of age with severe dysplasia in whom little capacity for remodeling remains. Dr. John Wilson has reported his experience with this procedure in a group of adolescents with very good results. It is not indicated in the younger child where a better alignment can be done. Fig. 8 demonstrates the level and manner in which a shelf procedure is to be performed.

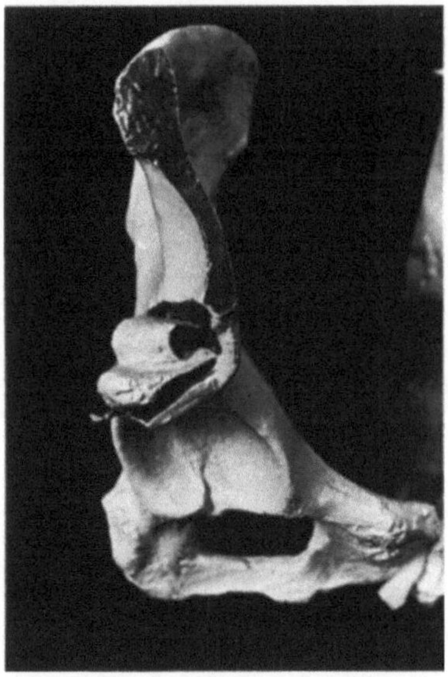

Fig. 8. Model demonstrates proper level at which shelf acetabuloplasty should be performed

Summary

In considering selection of one of the above osteotomies, one must have decided that the major problem lies on the acetabular side and that the femoral head will center on the abduction test.

With moderately severe dysplasia and an increased size of acetabulum, the Pemberton osteotomy may be performed providing sufficient growth potential remains to allow for acetabular remodeling. In the older child or adolescent with severe deformity, the Steel or Sutherland should be considered as a redirection-type osteotomy. In the adolescent with a dysplastic hip who needs only a stabilizing containment force, the properly performed shelf acetabuloplasty may be quite beneficial.

References

Coleman, S. S.: Clin. Orthop. **98,** 116 (1974)
Pemberton, P. A.: J. Bone Jt. Surg. **47A,** 65 (1965)
Pemberton, P. A.: Clin. Orthop. **98,** 41 (1974)
Steel, H. H.: J. Bone Jt. Surg. **55A,** 343 (1973)
Steel, H. H.: Clin. Orthop. **122,** 116 (1977)
Sutherland, D.: Personal Communication
Wilson, J. C., Jr.: Clin. Orthop. **98,** 137 (1974)

Skeletal Dysplasias in Childhood

Constitutional Disorders of Skeletal Development: The Skeletal Dysplasias

J. Spranger*

I. Definition and Classification

Constitutional disorders of skeletal development are inborn (primary) errors of skeletal growth and/or differentiation. They lead to abnormalities of skeletal form or structure called anomalies or malformations. Dwarfism is a major clinical manifestation of primary errors of skeletal development.

Constitutional disorders of skeletal development are differentiated from secondary bone disease in which the skeletal anlage, i.e., the primary growth and developmental potential of bone as tissue or organ, is normal. Abnormalities of skeletal form or structure caused by secondary bone diseases are called deformities.

Constitutional disorders of skeletal development are classifiable into hypo- and hyperplasias, dysostoses and dysplasias (Fig. 1).

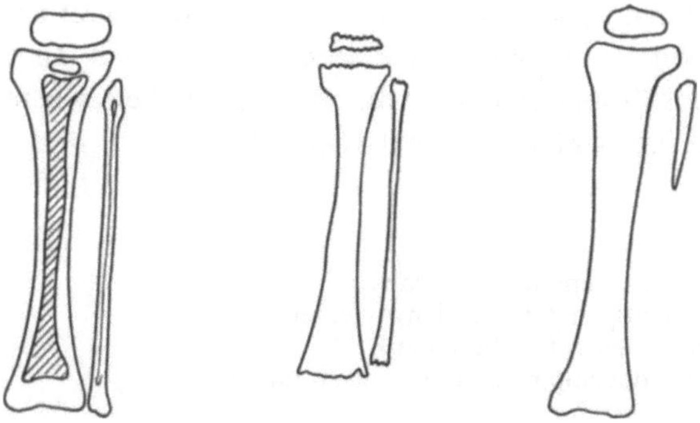

Fig. 1. Classification of constitutional errors of skeletal development

Skeletal hypo- and hyperplasias manifest themselves by change in size of one bony segment, several bony segments or the whole skeleton without change in the bone shape. They are caused by a deficiency or excess of number and/or size of cells constituting the skeletal system. Primordial shortness of stature is an example of generalized skeletal hypoplasia whereas the Marfan syndrome exemplifies a generalized hyperplasia.

* Children's Hospital University of Mainz, Federal Republic of Germany

Dysostoses are defined as congenital developmental anomalies of single bones, either solitary or in combination.

Phylogenetically they involve local organ, and not systemic tissue, defects. The lesions are mostly asymmetric and affect the shape of the bone more than the structure. They are divided into different groups according to their sites of predilection (Table 1).

Table 1. Morphological Classification of Dysostoses

Dysostoses with predominant involvement of the	
Neurocranium	(e.g., isolated craniostenosis; acrocephalosyndactyly)
Viscerocranium	(e.g., Dysostosis mandibulofacialis)
Axial skeleton	(e.g., Klippel-Feil syndrome)
Extremities	(e.g., Phocomelia)
Hands and Feet	(e.g., Polydactyly)

Skeletal dysplasias are systemic developmental anomalies of the cartilaginous and osseous tissues. They primarily involve not organ but tissue defects. For example, only epiphyseal ossification or only metaphyseal cartiliginous cell proliferation may be defective and the resulting epiphyseal or metaphyseal lesions would be predominantly symmetrical and would be distributed over an extensive part of the skeletal system. Multiple cartilaginous exostoses, for example, appear at the sites of rapid endochondral growth. Osteogenesis imperfecta is manifested primarily in sites of intramembranous bone formation. Due to developmental processes not yet fully understood, certain segments of the skeleton may be more affected than others, but always all similar structures are involved. Presently over 100 skeletal dysplasias have been well described. They can be divided into seven groups (Table 2) and are reported in detail elsewhere [1–3]. This survey is only concerned with the skeletal dysplasias.

Table 2. Classification of Skeletal Dysplasias

1. Skeletal dysplasias with predominantly epiphyseal involvement
2. Skeletal dysplasias with predominantly metaphyseal involvement
3. Skeletal dysplasias with major involvement of the spine
4. Skeletal dysplasias due to anarchic development of bone constituents
5. Osteolyses
6. Skeletal dysplasias with predominant involvement of single sites or segments
7. Skeletal dysplasias with abnormalities of bone density and/or modeling defects

II. Frequency

The total frequency of skeletal dysplasias is not known and is difficult to trace. The frequencies of some individual conditions are listed in Table 3. Since the number of different conditions is considerable [1] the incidence of skeletal dysplasias is estimated to be 1 in 1000.

The number of undetected cases is quite high for two reasons. Dominantly inherited dysplasias like osteogenesis imperfecta or epiphyseal dysplasia (Fairbank-Ribbing) can be present without clinical symptoms and may skip a generation ("reduced penetrance"). In a series of patients with hereditary arthro-ophthalmopathy (Stickler) epiphyseal dysplasia was manifest in only 25% [11]. Seventy-five per cent of the patients had the mutation, but it was not apparent in the skeleton.

Table 3. Frequency of Some Skeletal Dysplasias

Neonatally manifested skeletal dysplasias	~2.0:10,000 (4)
Multiple cartilaginous exostoses	~0.5:10,000 (5)
Osteogenesis imperfecta	~0.7:10,000 (6)
Mucopolysaccharidoses	~0.3:10,000 (7, 8)
Achondroplasia	~0.2:10,000 (9, 10)

The second reason for the presumably large number of undetected cases is false diagnosis. Only single symptoms are described, a local diagnosis is made and the essential systemic deficiency is overlooked. In a personally observed family with epiphyseal dysplasia (Fairbank-Ribbing) a whole array of diagnoses was made in various gene carriers, e.g., Scheuermann disease, spondylarthrosis, coxarthrosis, gonarthrosis, idiopathic hip dysplasia, bilateral Perthes disease, and rheumatoid arthritis. A correct diagnosis of Fairbank-Ribbing disease was reached in only one of the 14 affected individuals (Fig. 2).

III. Practical Aspects

Although no specific therapy for any skeletal dysplasia is yet available the practical importance of an exact diagnosis should not be underestimated for the following reasons:

The natural *course* is predictable if an exact diagnosis has been made. The child with severe autosomal recessive chondrodysplasia punctata will, in all probability, die before the end of the first year. In contrast, the prognosis for the autosomal dominant (Conradi-Hünermann) type is generally good. Although the patients later show epiphyseal defects, scoliosis and occasionally cataracts with skin and hair changes, their life expectancy and mental development are normal. Patients with epiphyseal dysplasias must expect considerable painful joint involvement later on and a sedentary occupation is recommended. Joint function remains unimpaired in metaphyseal chondrodysplasias.

Usually, the parents are concerned about the final stature of their children. With an exact diagnosis an empirical answer is possible. For example, patients with achondroplasia attain a height of up to 135 cm. Patients with morphologically similar hypochondroplasia, however, attain a height of up to 147 cm.

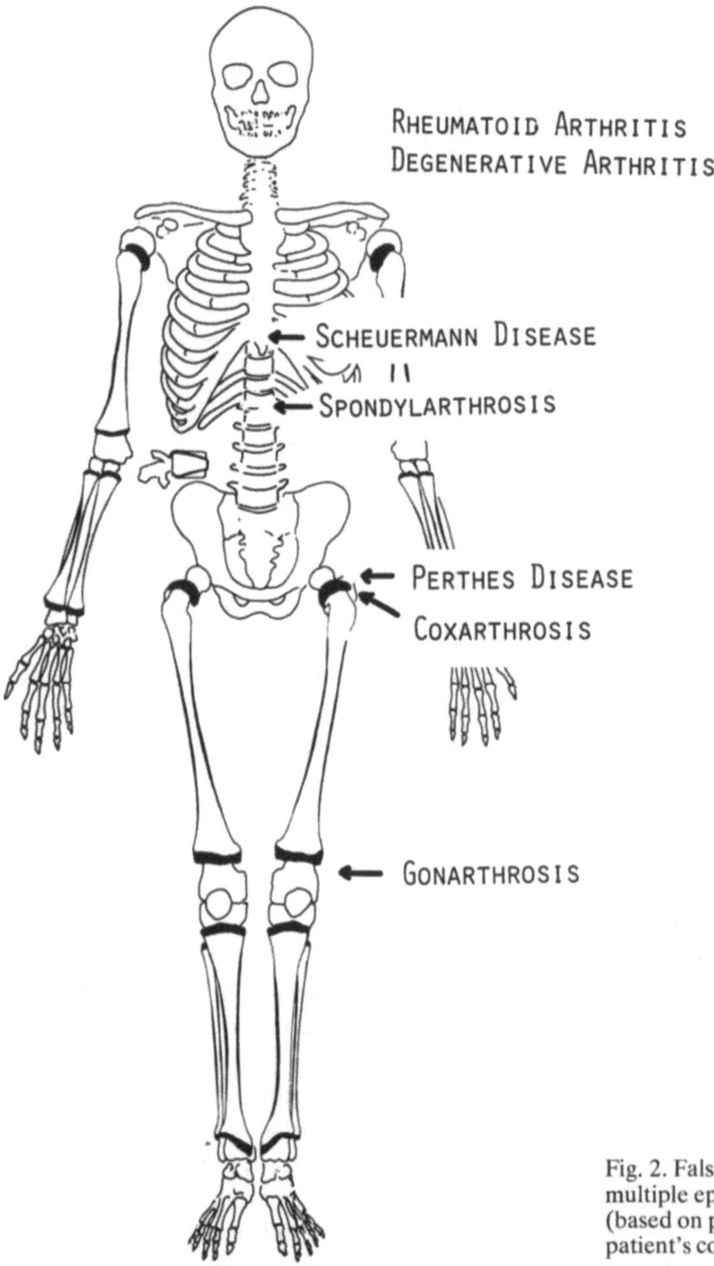

Fig. 2. False diagnoses in multiple epiphyseal dysplasia (based on principal sites of patient's complaints)

Complications can be avoided. An infant with metatropic dwarfism may not arouse suspicion. He will, however, inevitably develop a severe spinal deformity requiring early orthopaedic attention. Because of the laxity of the ligaments and hypoplasia of the odontoid process, atlantoaxial instability with threatening cervical cord compression may develop. Atlantoaxial instability has been observed in all skeletal dysplasias with platyspondyly and ligamentons laxity, especially in Morquio disease. In these disorders one has to look for neurologic

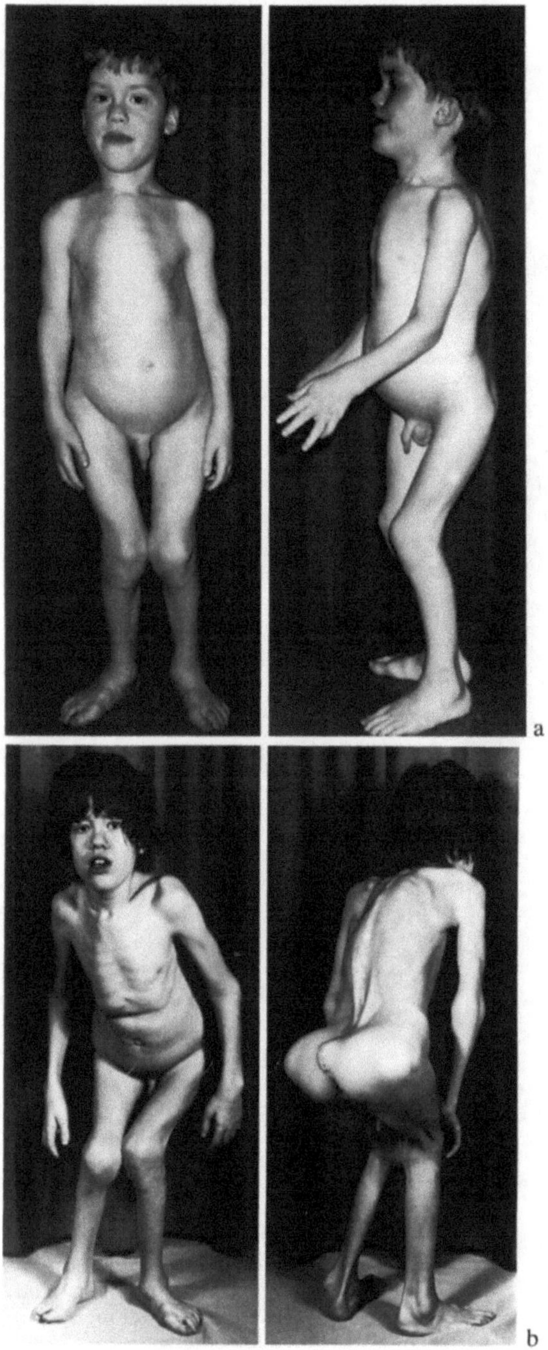

Fig. 3. Patient with metatropic dwarfism. (a) Age 4 years. (b). Age 9 years. There is a progressive kyphoscoliosis. Spastic tetraplegia developed after minor trauma due to atlantoaxial instability and cervical spinal cord compression. Severe secondary joint contractures

deficits as an indication for possible surgical fusion of the upper cervical segment [12]. Increased fatigue of the patient may be an early symptom.

Case S. T., at the age of 5, showed disproportionate short stature with a short neck, moderately severe kyphoscoliosis and flexion contractures of the hips, knees, and elbows. No neurologic deficits were noted (Fig. 3a). He suffered a mild injury at age 9 when he was thrown out of his seat as the result of a bus stopping suddenly. He then developed a

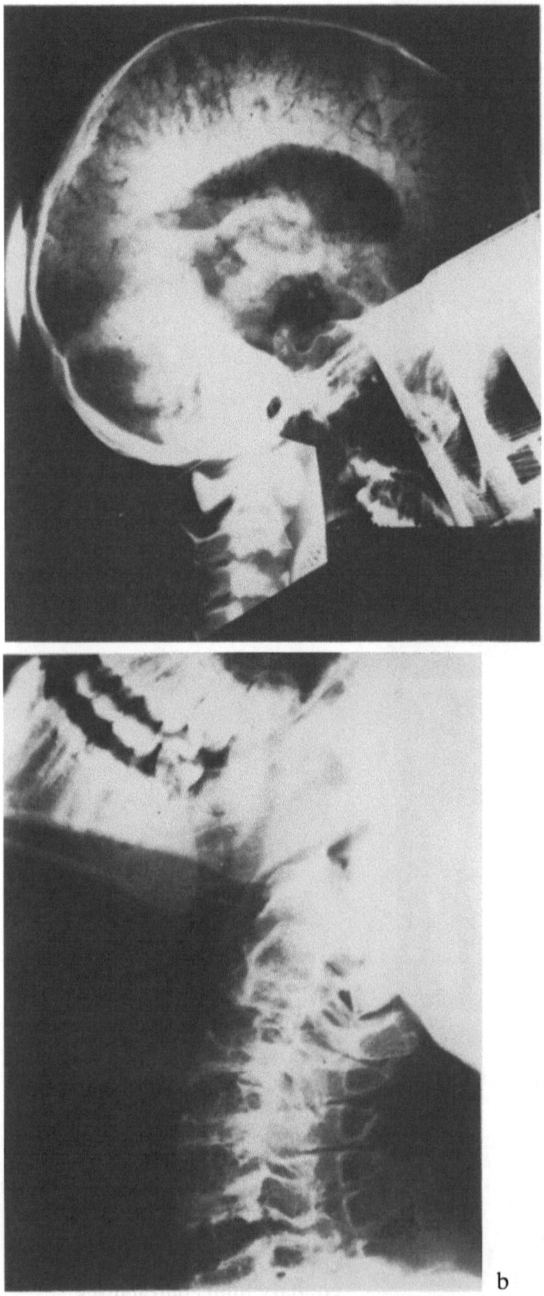

a

b

Fig. 4. Patient of Figure 3 at 9 years. There is moderate ventricular dilatation. The upper cervical bodies are dysplastic. Spinal decompression was performed. At operation, the first vertebra was seen to be displaced anteriorly with partial occlusion of the occipital foramen and marked compression of the medulla oblongata complete tetraplegia with respiratory difficulties. After several months of hospitalization his condition improved but increased joint contractures and a severe muscle atrophy developed. He complained of sensory changes, rapid fatigue and finally was scarcely able to walk. The tentative diagnosis was a possible progressive muscular dystrophy. On arrival at our hospital, he presented signs of transverse spinal compression with spastic tetraplegia and sensory deficits (Fig. 3 b). General and functional X-rays and tomography showed a horizontal gap of the odontoid process which originally was interpreted as a fracture, but which was possibly due to a congenital ossification anomaly. Myelography demonstrated a constricted cervical channel at the atlantoóccipital segment with moderate internal hydrocephalus (Fig. 4). We decided on surgical exploration of the upper cervical segment because of progressive neurologic deficits and on the basis of radiologically proven atlantoaxial instability which would have lead to further complications. The surgery revealed a displacement of the arch of the atlas into the occipital foramen with marked compression of the medulla oblongata which could be decompressed by resection of the atlas arch and widening of the intervertebral foramen followed by a dorsal fusion of the occipito – cervical region with autologous bone.

Skeletal dysplasias must be differentiated from the morphologically similar secondary developmental abnormalities of the cartilaginous-osseous system.

The differential diagnosis determines the choice of the therapeutic procedure. Some patients can be spared unnecessary and risky treatment. For instance, the use of thyroxine is not indicated in epiphyseal dysplasia but is necessary in radiographically similar hypothyroidism (Fig. 5). Metaphyseal structural changes are, for example, observed in metaphyseal chondrodysplasia, familial hypophosphatemic rickets, Menkes syndrome, scurvy and in battered children. The therapeutic procedures vary (Fig. 6, Table 4).

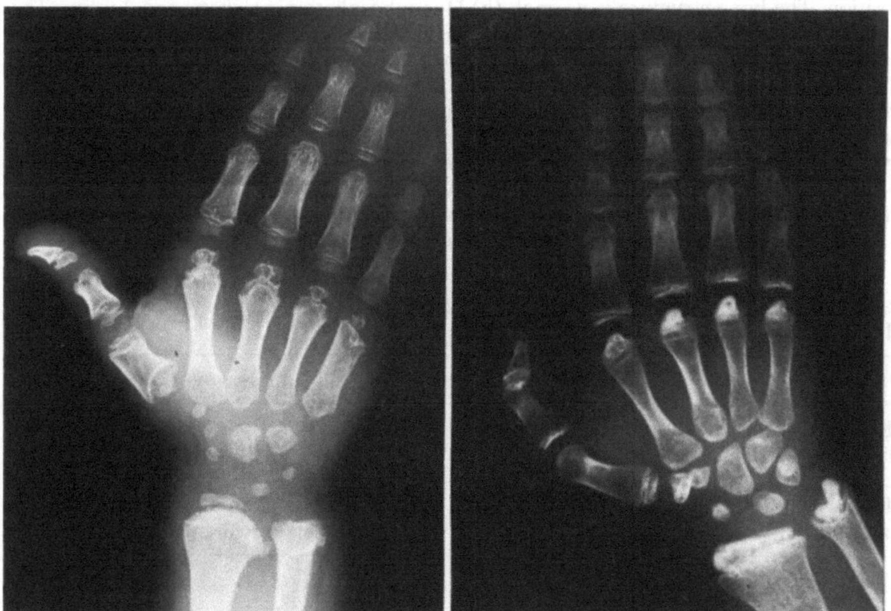

a b

Fig. 5. (a) Multiple epiphyseal dysplasia; age 9 years. The epiphyses and carpal bones are small and deformed. There are moderate metaphyseal irregularities of the distal forearms. (b) Untreated hypothyroidism; age 26 years. The epiphyses are small, irregular and densely ossified. The bone age is approximately 10 years

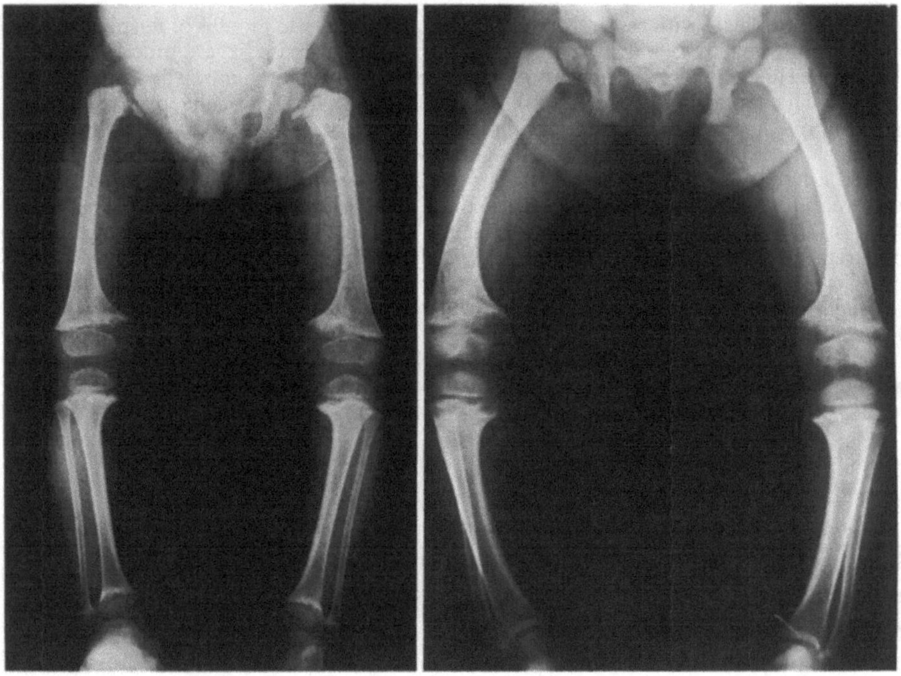

a b

Fig. 6. Metaphyseal abnormalities in five different conditions (Table 4). (a) Metaphyseal chondrodysplasia, Schmid type; age 2 years. The metaphyseal irregularities are more pronounced in the proximal than in the distal femora. The femoral necks are in varus position. The bone structure is normal. (b) Hypophosphatemic rickets; age 2 years. The metaphyseal irregularities are similar to those in Figure 6 a. The bone structure is, however, abnormal, and there is marked external bowing of the long bones due to osteomalacia. (c) Scurvy; age 10 months. There are mild metaphyseal irregularities. The ground-glass appearance with central radiolucency of the epiphyses (ring sign) and the metaphyseal fractures (corner sign) point to the correct diagnosis. (d) Menkes syndrome; age 10 months. The skeletal deformities in hereditary copper malabsorption are similar to those in scurvy but may also be confused with those in a battered child. (e) Battered child; age 9 months. The metaphyseal irregularities are caused by avulsion fractures at the sites of ligamentous and/or periosteal attachment to bone

Table 4. Differential therapy of five disorders with distinct metaphyseal irregularities (depicted in Fig. 6 a–e)

Diagnosis	*Therapy*
Metaphyseal chondrodysplasia, Schmid type	No medical therapy
Hypophosphatemic rickets	Vitamin D and phosphate
Scurvy	Vitamin C
Menkes syndrome	Copper infusions?
Battered child	Social measures

Finally, *genetic counseling* depends on an exact diagnosis. With healthy parents it is unlikely that achondroplasia would recur but if one parent is affected there is a 50% chance of this condition recurring. The recurrence risk amounts to 25% in autosomal recessive conditions. An incomplete diagnosis can have disastrous consequences as the following case illustrates.

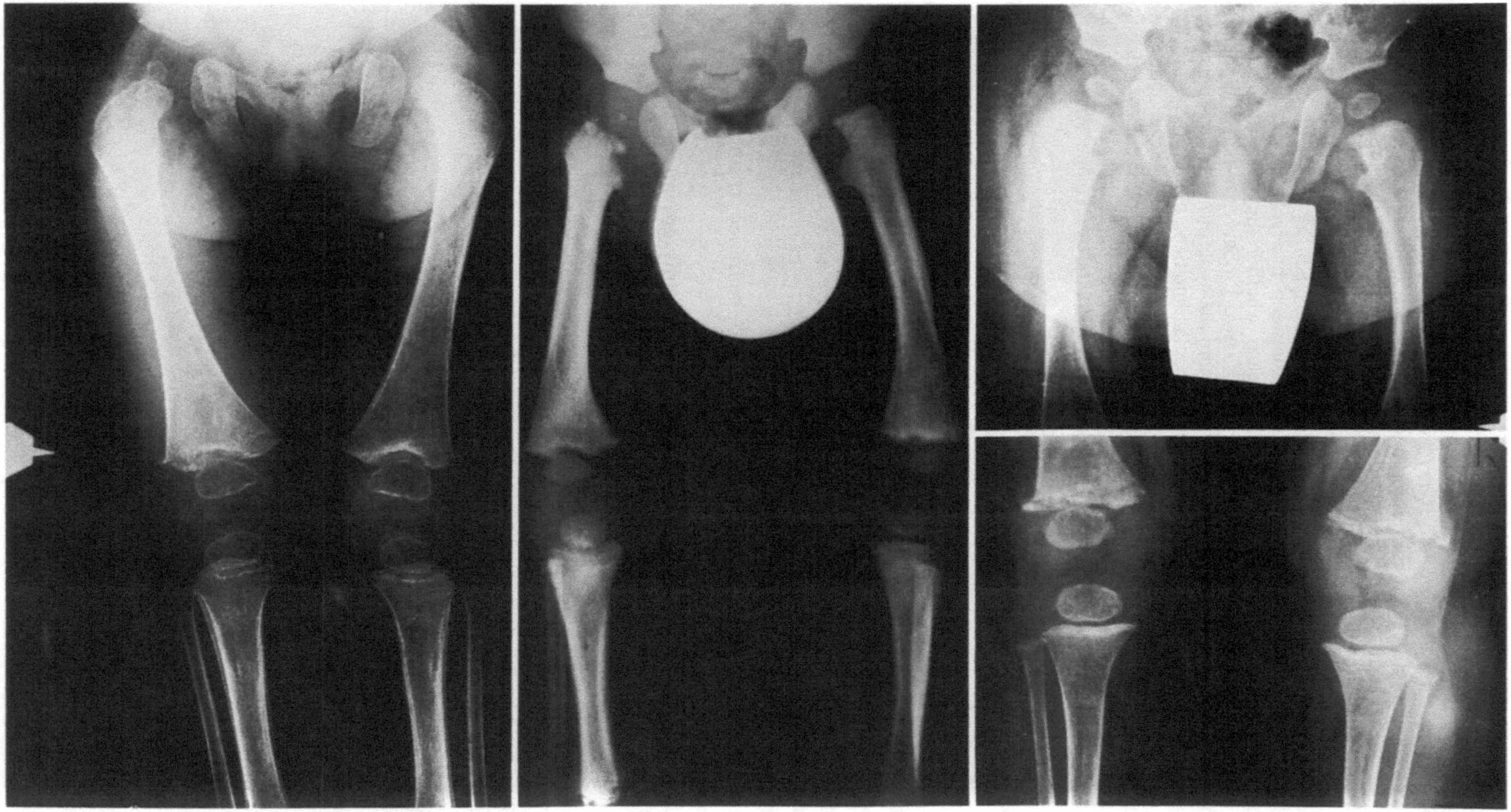

c d e

Fig. 6c–e

Patient A. B., the first child of young, nonconsanguineous parents, died shortly after birth. His height was 37 cm. No X-ray examination was carried out. The autopsy and pathology reports revealed shortening and cartilaginous distention of the ends of the tubular bones. Histologically, the proliferation zones of the growth plate were irregular with total lack of columnar formation, and increased amounts of resting cartilage. The parents were concerned about the possibility of the disease occurring in future children when the diagnosis of hyperplastic chondrodysplasia was made.

Since 1893 pathologists have differentiated between hyperplastic and hypoplastic chondrodystrophy [13]. It has never become clear whether they were thought of as varieties of one genopathy or two separate diseases. Probably so-called hypoplastic chondrodystrophy is identical to achondroplasia and the hyperplastic form is metatropic dwarfism. Achondroplasia is inherited as an autosomal dominant, metatropic dwarfism in the severe expression, as an autosomal recessive. In the described case, achondroplasia could be ruled out on clinical grounds. However, without more specific data, a definite diagnosis was not possible and thus made genetic counseling impossible. In all probability, a single X-ray examination would have helped to make the exact diagnosis.

IV. Diagnostic Procedures

Generally one must consider the possibility of a skeletal dysplasia when the patient presents with:

Reduced growth

Positive family history

Symmetrically extensive skeletal changes

Atypical course of an orthopaedic condition

Presence of dysmorphic stigmata (different appearance from other family members)

For diagnosis, roentgenograms of a series of rapidly growing and diagnostically relevant skeletal regions are necessary. We recommend lateral films of the spine and a-p views of the pelvis and hands. If no abnormalities are found in these areas a skeletal dysplasia is unlikely. If abnormal changes are found, however, further examination of other bony segments is necessary for an exact diagnosis (Table 5). Though distinct skeletal abnormalities are present in many bone dysplasias they are rarely specific for a single condition. The diagnosis of a bone

Table 5. X-ray program for suspected case of skeletal dysplasia

A. Screening
1. Lateral view of lower thoracic and lumbar spine
2. A-p. view of pelvis
3. Hands

B. Full program
4. Knees and shanks a-p
5. Lateral skull
6. A-p. thorax
7. A-p. elbow and forearm
8. A-p. humerus and femur

C. Search for characteristic findings in selected dysplasias
i. e., Wormian bones in osteogenesis imperfecta
i. e., craniocaudal narrowing of lumbar interpedicular distance in achondroplasia
i. e., short metacarpals in pseudohypoparathyroidism

dysplasia must be based on the total pattern of anomalies, not on single signs. Recourse to atlases of dysplasias and registers in various dysplasia centers are helpful in making the diagnosis.

V. Examples

As an introduction to the sometimes bewildering field of bone dysplasias, a few conditions will be illustrated. They belong to groups 1–3 of Table 2, i.e., disorders caused by defects of endochondral bone formation. Detailed reviews are available [1–3].

Dysplasia Epiphysealis Multiplex (Ribbing disease, Fairbank disease)

The mild form of epiphyseal dysplasia was described by Ribbing in 1937 in a large family [14]. In this type of dysplasia the proximal femoral epiphyses are flattened and the condition has been labeled as "flat type" of epiphyseal dys-

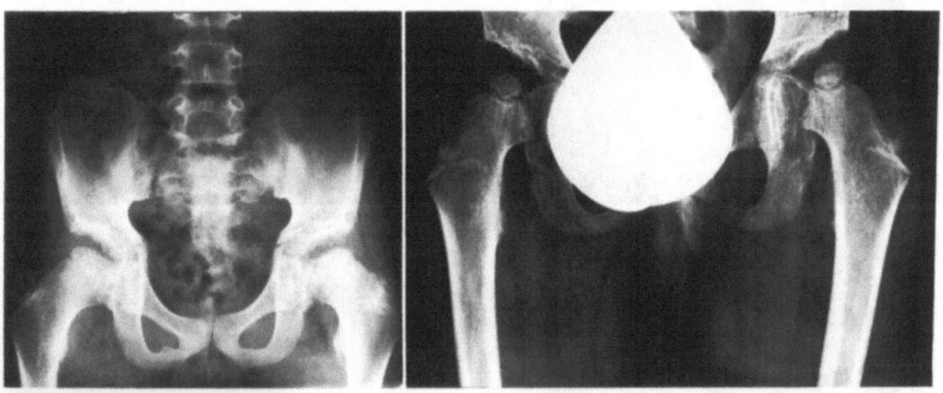

a b

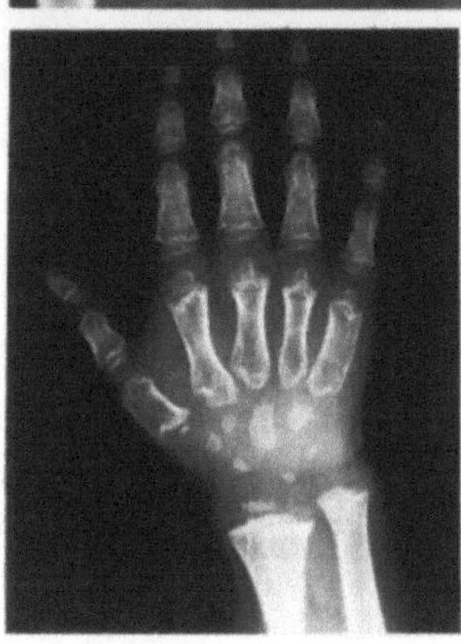

c

Fig. 7. (a) Multiple epiphyseal dysplasia, Ribbing type; age 14 years. The capital femoral epiphyses are flattened and their contours are slightly irregular; the lower portions of the ilia are broad. (b) Multiple epiphyseal dysplasia, Fairbank type; age 8 years. The capital femoral epiphyses are small and the acetabular roofs are irregular with a wide acetabular angle. (c) Multiple epiphyseal dysplasia Fairbank type; age 5 years. The epiphyses and carpal bones are small and their contours are irregular. The tubular bones are short with slightly irregular metaphyseal margins plasia [15]. The severe form of epiphyseal dysplasia was thoroughly investigated by Fairbank [16]. Due to the deformity of the proximal femoral epiphysis the condition was labeled as the "microepiphysis" type of multiple epiphyseal dysplasia [15]. It has not been determined as yet whether the mild (Ribbing) type and the severe (Fairbank) type are variable manifestations of one disease or are etiologically different disorders. Both forms are inherited as an autosomal dominant. In the severe cases, joint pain, back pain, and a waddling gait appear in early childhood. Patients with the mild form experience these symptoms only in later life. Radiologically, deformed epiphyseal centers in the hip, knee and ankle joints, and hands appear in childhood. In adults the joint surfaces are deformed by cysts and secondary diminution of the joint spaces (Fig. 7). The prognosis depends on the degree of involvement of the epiphyseal ossification centers. Severe arthrotic changes sometimes appear in the third decade of life, but mostly occur later. Prophylactically, sedentary occupations and sports or swimming are recommended. In therapy, prosthetic replacement of the hip or, more rarely, the knee joints have to be considered sooner or later.

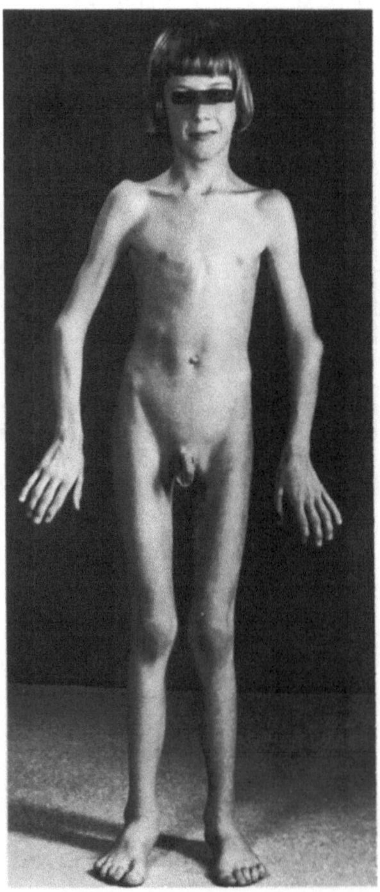

a

Fig. 8. (a and b) Stickler syndrome (hereditary arthroophthalmopathy). The extremities are long and thin. The capital femoral epiphyses are flat and deformed, the femoral necks are wide. There is but little iliac flare

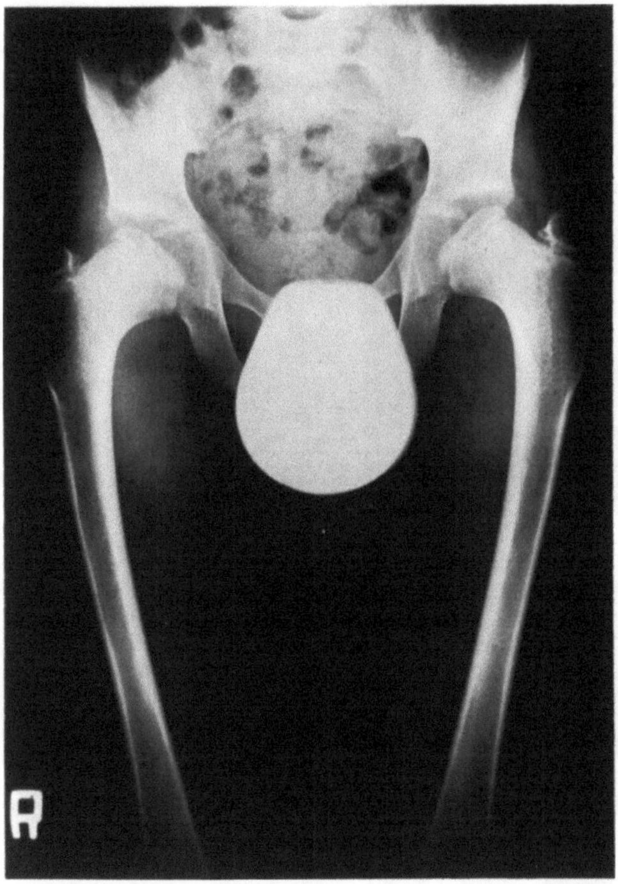

Fig. 8b

The most frequent misdiagnoses are "multiple arthrosis" and "osteochondrosis." Symmetrical involvement of several joints, familial occurrence and – in contrast to osteochondroses – progressive destruction of the epiphyseal center without signs of regeneration, indicate the correct diagnosis.

Special Forms of Epiphyseal Dysplasias

Localized epiphyseal disorders are most frequently found in the capital femoral epiphyses. Meyer has differentiated an isolated epiphyseal dysplasia of the femoral head from bilateral Perthes disease [17]. It appears to be transmitted as an autosomal dominant. Occasionally epiphyseal changes are restricted to the spine and the knee or elbow joints. Thiemann disease [18] may be considered as a localized epiphyseal dysplasia of the fingers.

In patients with eye diseases (myopia, retinal detachment, cataracts, loss of eye sight) and early arthrosis the syndrome described by Stickler as hereditary arthroophthalmopathy has to be considered [11]. These patients are slim with a Marfan-type habitus and have multiple epiphyseal anomalies (Fig. 8).

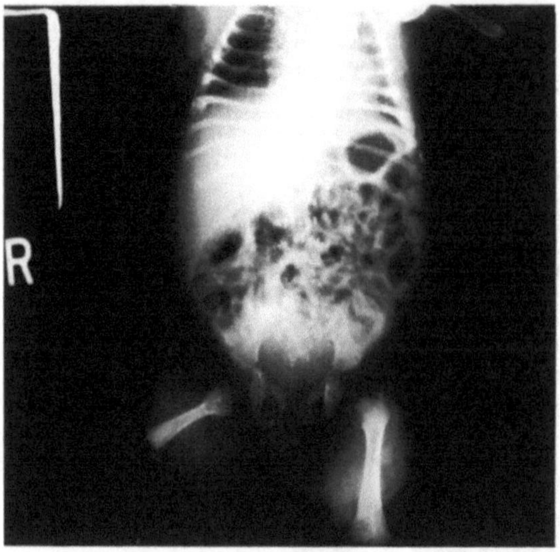

a

b

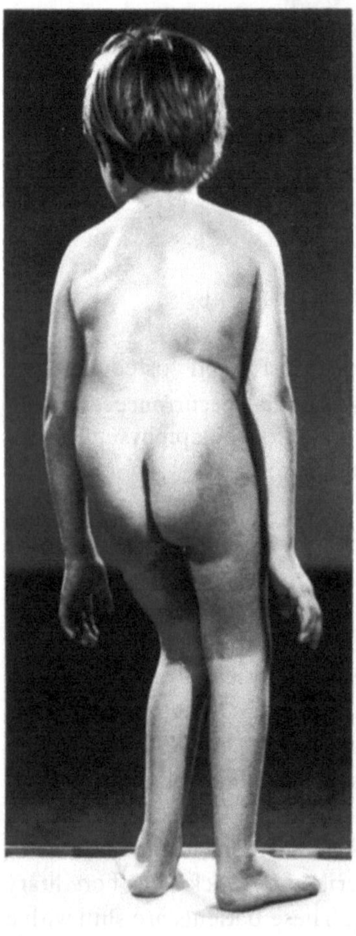

Fig. 9. Chondrodysplasia punctata, Conradi-Hünermann type. (a) Newborn. The right femur is shorter than the left. There are numerous calcific stipples in the right hip and knee region and along the spine. (b) Age 6 years. There is a marked kyphoscoliosis. The right leg is shortened. (c) Age 4 years. The ossification of the left capital femoral epiphysis is retarded and multicentric. Earlier calcifications in this region have disappeared

c

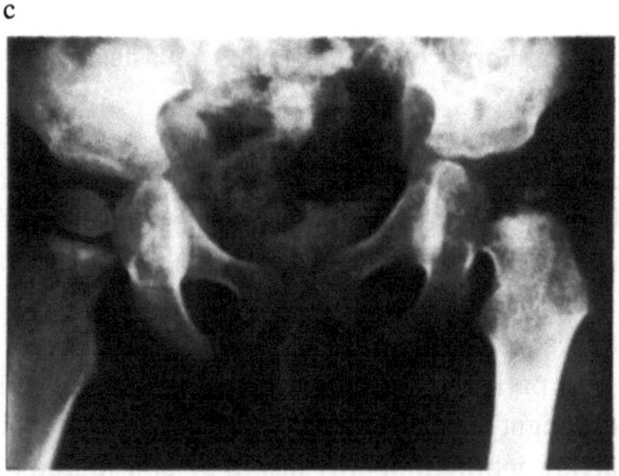

Asymmetric ossification anomalies of the epiphyseal centers, frequently with severe spinal curvature, arouse suspicion of chondrodysplasia punctata (Conradi-Hünermann type). The calcific spots in the epiphyseal and periarticular areas, which are typical for this disorder, are found only in infants. The presence of frequently asymmetrically distributed epiphyseal deformities and scoliosis suggest the diagnosis at a later age (Fig. 9). Clinical symptoms include scoliosis, asymmetric limb shortening ichthyotic skin changes, partial alopecia, and cataracts. However, not all clinical changes are present in every patient. In addition to treatment of the scoliosis, lengthening procedures of the lower extremity must be considered in the presence of unilateral leg shortening.

Achondroplasia

Achondroplasia is the best known of the generalized skeletal dysplasias. Histologically there is evidence of retarded enchondral cartilaginous cell proliferation as the cartilage cell colums are shortened. Epiphyseal ossification and thus joint development and function are normal. Of special orthopaedic interest are the varus deformities of the lower legs (Fig. 10). The fibula is comparatively less shortened than the tibia. Braces are not recommended in the varus deformities because of the prominent fibular head with danger of peroneal nerve compression and the shortened and thickened lower limbs [19]. Correction osteotomies are rarely indicated since the malposition, particularly of the ankle joint, is well tolerated without essential functional deficits and later complications. If difficulties with footwear and cosmetic demands should necessitate osteotomy, Outland's method is recommended [19].

Occasionally adults with achondroplasia show anterior wedging of one or several vertebral bodies with kyphosis and possible constriction of the spinal canal at the thoracolumbar level. Sensory changes of the lower extremities with possible bladder involvement represent early symptoms of spinal cord compression necessitating myelography and possibly surgery.

Larsen Syndrome (Multiple Congenital Dislocations and Facial Dysmorphism)

This syndrome, extensively described by Larsen in 1950 [20], and known of before [e.g., 21, 22], is well-known to the orthopaedic surgeon. At birth multiple dislocations are noticed, particularly in the knee and hip joints, in addition to the typical facial anomaly (retracted, broad nasal base with high, arched forehead, Fig. 11a, b) and occasionally clubfeet and cleft palate. During its course typical skeletal changes appear which are not caused by dislocation but represent dysplastic skeletal development (Fig. 11c, d).

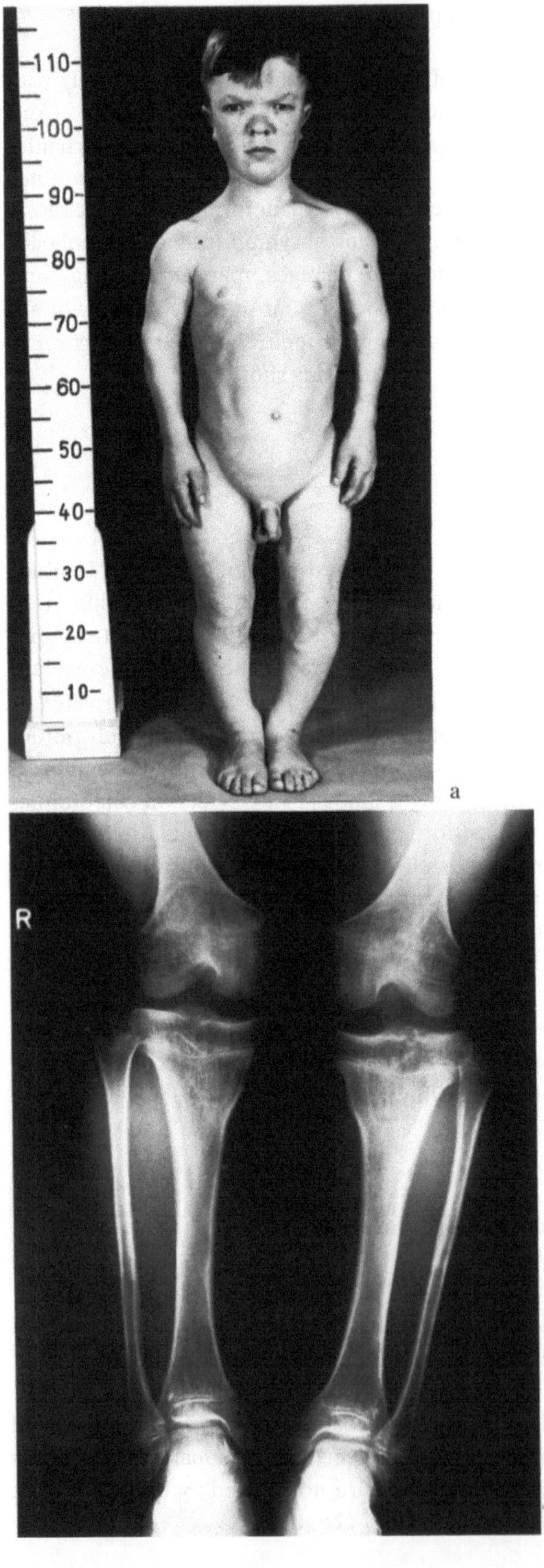

Fig. 10. Achondroplasia; age 10 years. (a) There is a long-trunk type of dwarfism. Crura vara. (b) The tibiae are short and broad with disproportionately long fibulae. The lateral portions of the distal femoral epiphyses are flattened

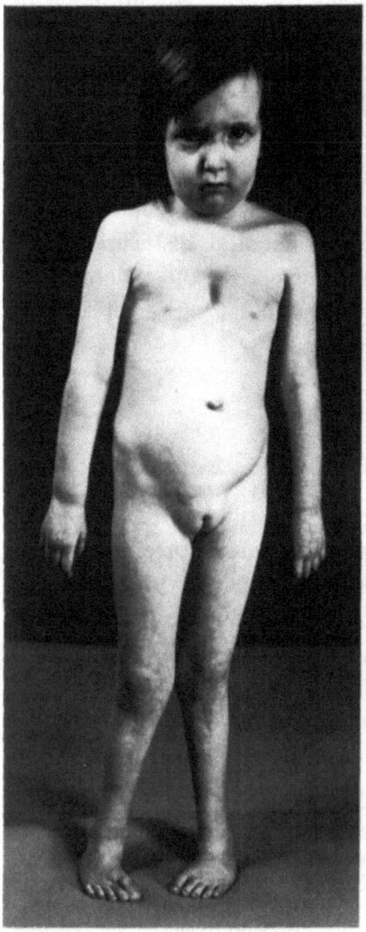

a

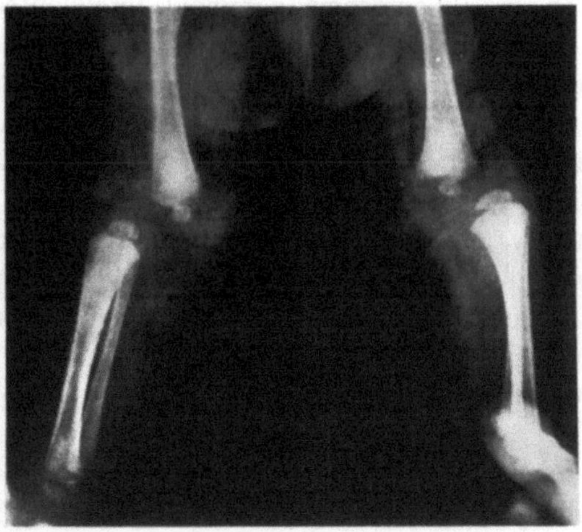

b

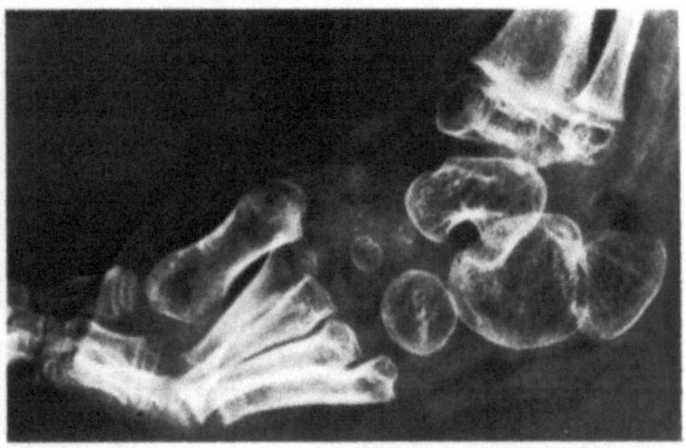

c

d

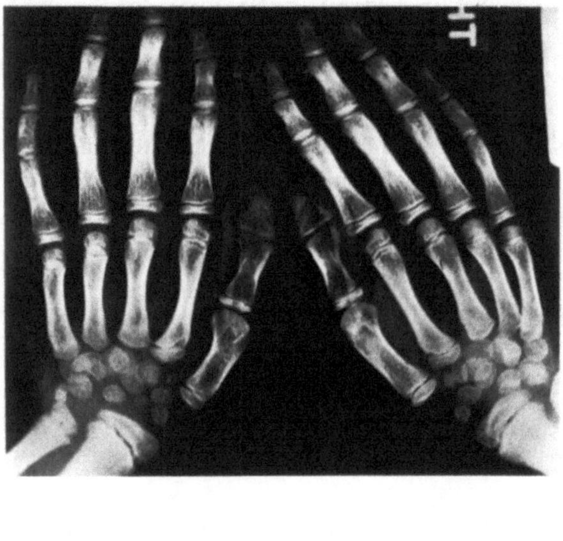

Fig. 11. Larsen syndrome. (a) Age 4 years. The nasal bridge is depressed, the forehead is prominent and there are multiple congenital dislocations. (b) Newborn. The tibiae and fibulae are dislocated anteriorly and laterally. (c) Age 4 years. Two calcaneal ossification centers are seen. The extra ossification center usually appears after the first year of life and usually fuses with the regular center after the fifth year. There are multiple dislocations. The bones are porotic. (d) Age 5 years. There are supernumerous carpal ossification centers. The distal ends of the first metacarpal, the proximal and the middle phalanges are wide and the distal phalanx of the thumb is short

The mostly autosomal dominant, rarely autosomal recessive condition has to be differentiated particularly from arthrogryposis multiplex. Both disorders, in the later stages, show contractures as well as dislocations. In arthrogryposis the contractures appear first with later dislocations; a reverse sequence occurs in Larsen syndrome. In Larsen syndrome, typical facial and dysplastic skeletal changes, especially in the hands, are seen; in arthrogryposis, periarticular atrophy, increased turgor and degenerative histologic muscular changes are the distinctive features. Other forms with multiple congenital dislocations are diastrophic dwarfism [1], Ehlers-Danlos syndrome [23], oto-palatodigital syndrome [1], and a peculiar dysplasia recently described by French authors [24].

Spondyloepiphyseal Dysplasias

These dysplasias show distinct and usually progressive changes of the epiphyses and vertebral bodies. Clinically, there is disproportionate shortening of the trunk. Of the numerous types of spondyloepiphyseal dysplasias three clinically similar and frequently misdiagnosed, but radiologically, genetically, and prognostically entirely different, well-defined types are depicted in Figures 12–14 and Table 6.

Table 6. Differential diagnosis of three frequently confused spondyloepiphyseal dysplasias

	Spondyloepiphyseal dysplasia congenita	Morquio disease (Mucopolysacchari-dosis type IV)	Spondyloepiphyseal dysplasia tarda
Manifestation	Birth	Second year	School age
Eyes	Myopia, retinal rents	Corneal opacities	Normal
Femoral neck	Varus	Valgus	Normal
Hands	No dysplasia	Severe dysplasia	Normal
Keratansulfaturia	No	Yes (in children)	No
Inheritance	Autosomal dominant	Autosomal recessive	X-chromosomal recessive

Spondyloepiphyseal Dysplasia Congenita has been differentiated in 1970 from Morquio disease [25]. It is an autosomal dominant disease while Morquio disease is transmitted as an autosomal recessive trait. The patients are small at birth and occasionally have clubfeet and cleft palates. Skeletal abnormalities include retarded ossification of the pubic bones and vertebrae. Later clinical changes are a short neck, short trunk, pectus carinatum (pigeon chest), lumbar hyperlordosis and genua valga.

Not infrequently myopia with possible retinal detachment but clear corneae are observed. Radiologically, the vertebral bodies are flat. The proximal epiphysis and femoral neck show late or no ossification so that plain films show

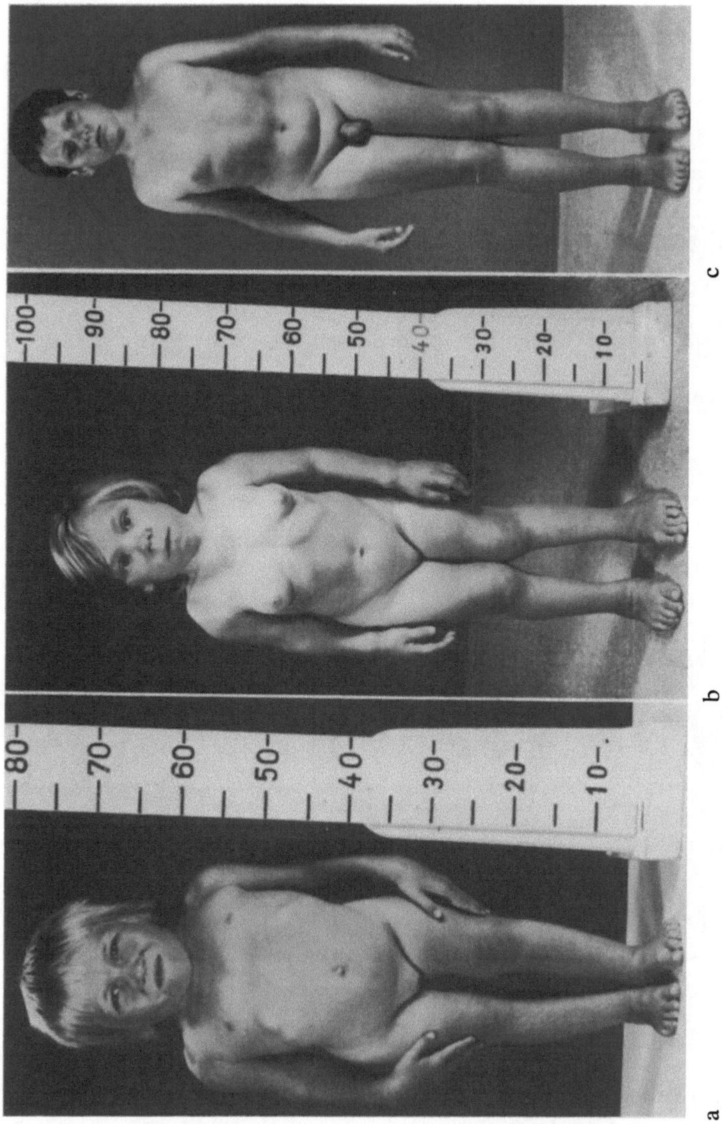

Fig. 12. Differential diagnosis of spondyloepiphyseal dysplasias. (a) Spondyloepiphyseal dysplasia congenita; age 5 years. (b) Morquio disease; age 6 years. The clinical appearance of Morquio disease and spondyloepiphyseal dysplasia congenita is similar but in Morquio disease the hands and fingers are short. (c) Spondyloepiphyseal dysplasia tarda; age 8 years. The trunk is moderately short

empty hip sockets (Fig. 15). The unossified femoral necks are in severe varus position. There is only scanty experience with respect to the prognosis of valgus osteotomy for correction of this marked varus deformity of the femoral necks. Regular ophthalmological follow-up and preventive treatment of peripheral retinal detachment can avoid possible later blindness.

Morquio disease is one of the seven well-defined mucopolysaccharidoses and is very rare. It has frequently been misdiagnosed but the pattern of X-ray findings is pathognomonic. One of the major clinical criteria is the presence of corneal opacities demonstrable by slit lamp microscopy. Keratan sulfate is present in the urine of children with Morquio disease but not always in adults.

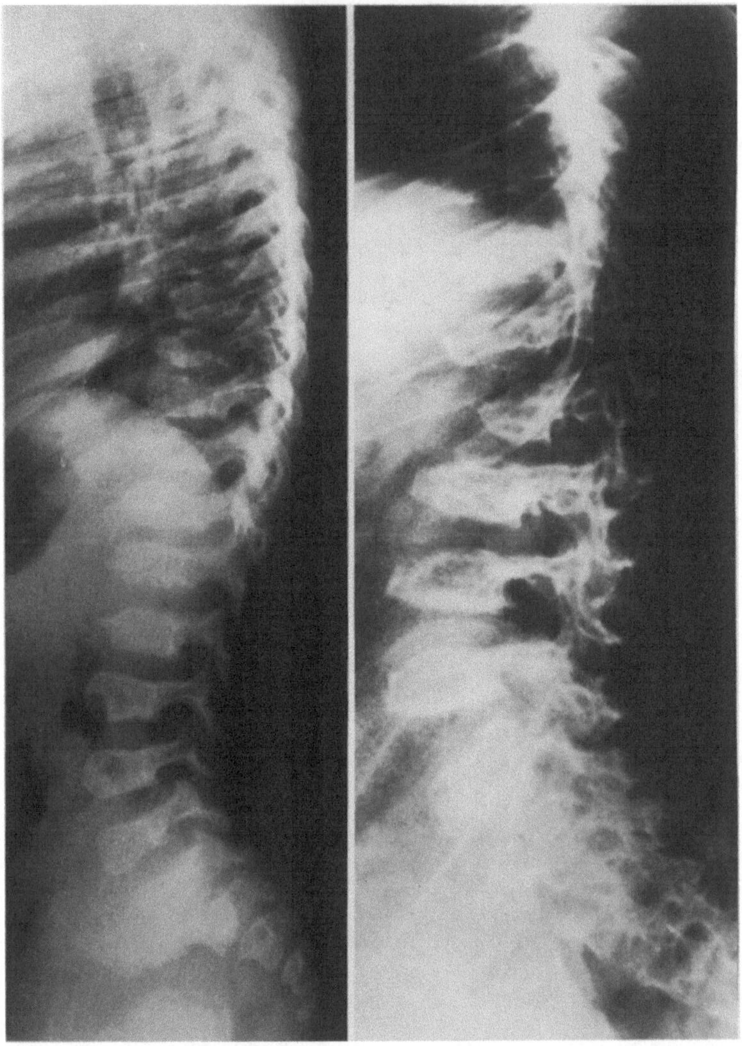

a b

Fig. 13 a and b

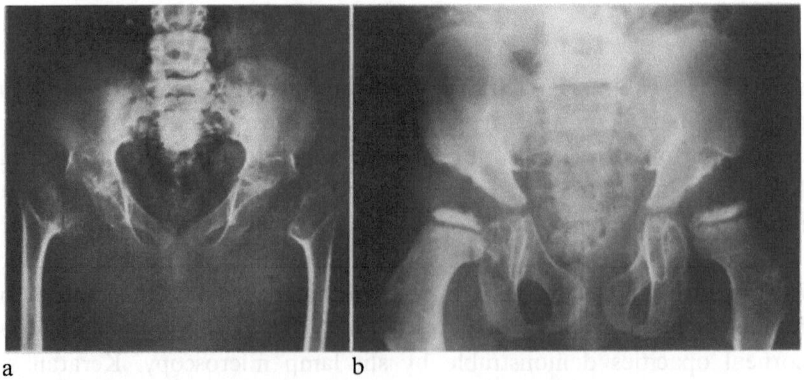

a b

Fig. 14 a and b

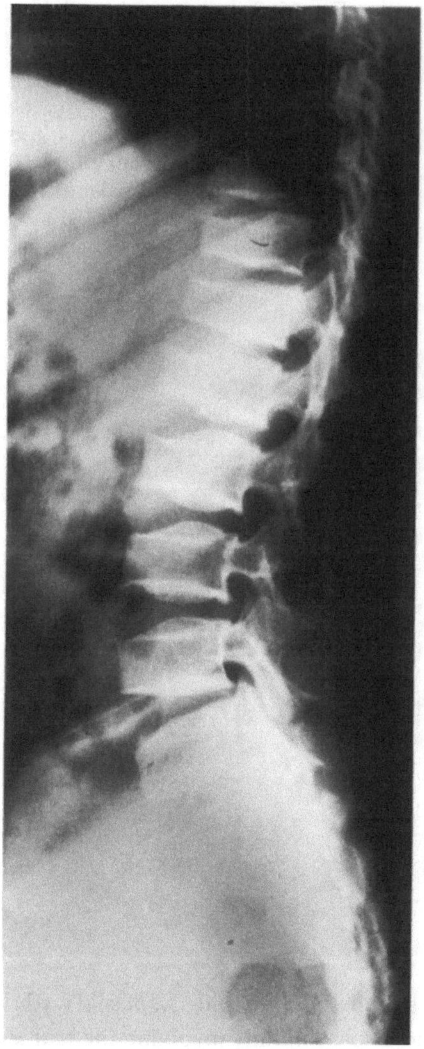

c

Fig. 13. Differential diagnosis of spondyloepiphyseal dysplasias. (a) Spondyloepiphyseal dysplasia congenita; age 5 years. There is dorsal wedging and anterior pointing of the vertebral bodies. (b) Morquio disease; age 11 years. The vertebral bodies are flat with anterior hypoplasia and retroposition of L-1. (c) Spondyloepiphyseal dysplasia tarda; age 10 years. The vertebral bodies are deformed with a characteristic hump-shaped build-up of bone in the central and posterior portions of the upper and lower plates

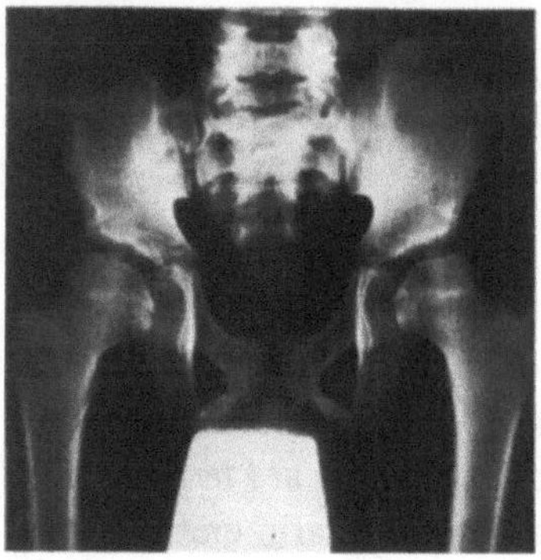

c

Fig. 14. Differential diagnosis of spondyloepiphyseal dysplasias. (a) Spondyloepiphyseal dysplasia congenita; age 13 years. The proximal femoral epiphysis and the neck are separated by a cartilaginous cleft. The femoral neck is in marked varus position. (b) Morquio disease; age 10 years. The femoral necks are in valgus position, the femoral epiphyses are flat and deformed and the inferior portions of the ilia are hypoplastic. (c) Spondyloepiphyseal dysplasia tarda; age 10 years. There is mild flattening of the proximal femoral epiphyses

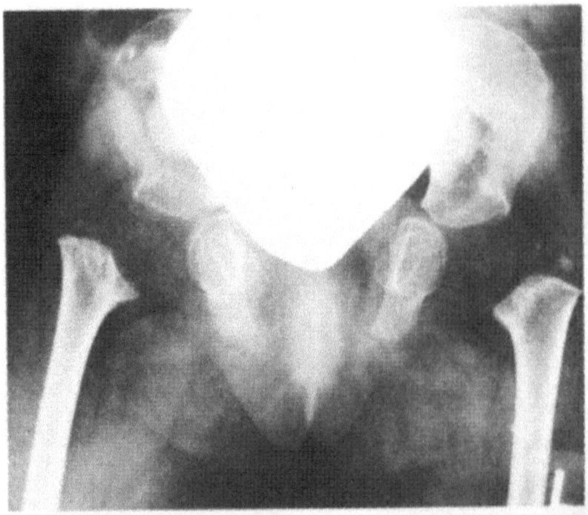

a

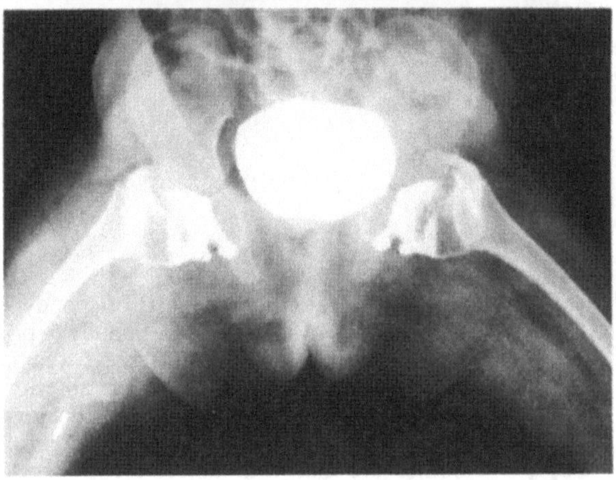

b

Fig. 15. Spondyloepiphyseal dysplasia congenita; age 3 years. (a) A plain film shows absent ossification of the femoral head and neck. The appearance may be misinterpreted as femoral dislocation. (b) Arthrography reveals a normal cartilage anlage of the femoral head and neck

The X-chromosomal recessive form of spondyloepiphyseal dysplasia tarda represents, in comparison, a mild form of the disease mainly involving the trunk and becoming manifest only between the ages of 6 and 12. According to inheritance, only boys are affected; the vertebral deformities are characteristic (Fig. 13c).

VI. Etiology and Pathogenesis

Bone dysplasias are caused by single gene mutations. Their skeletal manifestations may be mimicked by secondary bone diseases in which extraosseous factors disturb the development of primarily normal bones. Examples are hypothyroidism leading to a marked epiphyseal dysplasia (Fig. 5) or warfarin embryopathy copying the phenotype of chondrodysplasia punctata [26].

Table 7. Disorders of complex carbohydrate metabolism

Name	Synonym	Enzyme defect	Age at manifestation	X-ray: Dysostosis multiplex
Mucopolysaccharidosis I-H	Hurler disease	α-Iduronidase	Infancy	Severe
Mucopolysaccharidosis I-S	Scheie disease	α-Iduronidase	Late childhood	Mild
Mucopolysaccharidosis II	Hunter	Sulfaiduronate sulfatase	Late infancy	Moderate
Mucopolysaccharidosis III	Sanfilippo	Heparin sulfamidase α-Glucosaminidase	Early childhood	Mild
Mucopolysaccharidosis IV	Morquio	Chondroitin-6-sulfate sulfatase	Early childhood	Characteristic
Mucopolysaccharidosis VI	Maroteaux-Lamy	Chondroitin-4-sulfate sulfatase	Early childhood	Moderate
Mucopolysaccharidosis VII		α-Glucuronidase	Early childhood	Moderate
Mucolipidosis I		α-Neuraminidase	Midchildhood	Moderate
Mucolipidosis II	I-cell disease	Multiple lysosomal enzymes	Infancy	Severe
Mucolipidosis III	Pseudopolydystrophy	Multiple lysosomal enzymes	Early childhood	Characteristic
β-Galactosidase deficiency	G_{M_1}gangliosidosis	β-Galactosidase	Varying according to type	Varying according to type
Mannosidosis		α-Mannosidase	Early childhood	Mild
Fucosidosis		α-Fucosidase	Varying according to type	Minimal
Sandhoff disease	G_{M_2}gangliosidosis O-type	Hexosaminidases A & B	Infancy	Minimal
Aspartylglucosaminuria		Aspartylglucosamidohydrolase	Early childhood	Mild
Mucosulfatidosis	Austin variant of metachromatic leucodystrophy	Multiple sulfatases	Late infancy	Moderate

Chromosomal abnormalities, chemical, mechanical, hormonal or other intrauterine injuries to the fetus are more likely to result in dysostoses or skeletal hypoplasias than in dysplasias.

The pathogenesis of most bone dysplasias remains unknown in spite of major recent advances in their histologic delineation [27]. Exceptions are some inborn errors of metabolism known to be associated with bone dysplasias such as hypophosphatasia or disorders of complex carbohydrates. The latter lead to a characteristic pattern of bony anomalies called "dysostosis multiplex" (Fig. 16). Though much has been learned about the molecular basis of these disorders (Table 7), only few efforts have been made to explain the genesis of the peculiar bony abnormalities. One exception is the work of Ponseti on Morquio disease [28]. Apparently, in this disorder those cartilage sites are preferentially affected which are rich in large collagen bundles such as tendon and ligamentous insertions into cartilage. It has been speculated that keratan sulfate, which cannot be properly degraded in Morquio disease, abounds in these sites. Combining his observations regarding metabolism and histology with mechanical considerations, Ponseti was able to advance a unifying concept explaining the peculiar development of the skeleton in Morquio disease.

It is through this approach – the combination of clinical, biochemical, histological, and mechanical considerations – that future research will elucidate the nature of many of the theoretically fascinating but in practice sometimes bewildering disorders of skeletal development.

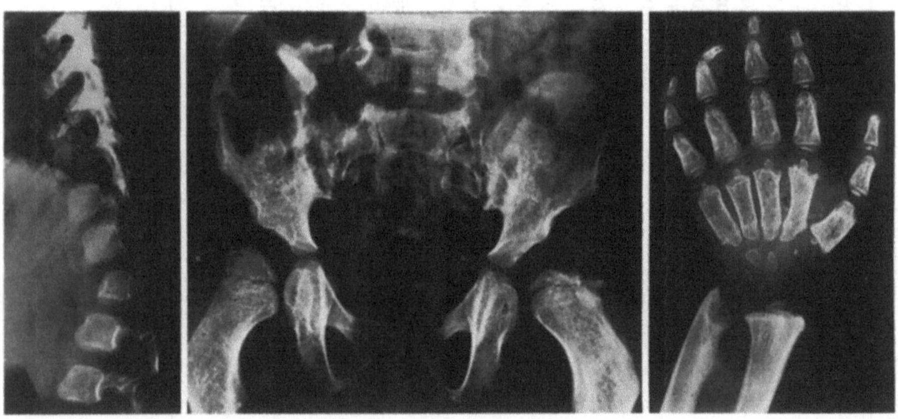

Fig. 16. Severe manifestation of dysostosis multiplex. The vertebrae are hookshaped. There is a characteristic pelvic dysplasia with notable underdevelopment of the inferior ilia. The femoral necks are in valgus position and the capital femoral epiphyses are deformed. The phalanges are bullet-shaped, the metacarpals are proximally pointed; the carpal bones and epiphyses are small and deformed

References

1. Spranger, J., Langer, L. O., Wiedemann, H. R.: Bone Dysplasias An Atlas of Constitutional Disorders of Skeletal Development. Stuttgart/Philadelphia: Fischer/ Saunders 1974
2. Maroteaux, P.: Maladies osseuses de l'enfant. Paris: Flammarion 1974
3. Rimoin, D. L.; ed.: Skeletal Dysplasias, Clin. Orthop. **114,** 1976
4. Harris, R., Patton, J. T.: Achondroplasia and thanatophoric dwarfism in the newborn. Clin. Genet. **2,** 61 1971
5. Murken, J. D.: Über multiple cartilaginäre Exostosen. Z. Menschl. Vererb. Konst.-lehre **36,** 460 (1963)
6. Schröder, G. O.: Osteogenesis imperfecta. Z. Menschl. Vererb. Konstit.lehre **37,** 632 1964
7. Lowry, R. B., Renwick, D. H. G.: Relative frequency of the Hurler and Hunter Syndromes. New Engl. J. Med. **284,** 221 1971
8. Spranger, J.: The Genetic Mucopolysaccharidoses. Ergebn. inn. Med. Kinderheilk. **32,** 165 1972
9. Schiemann, H.: Über Chondrodystrophie. Akd. Wissensch. Lit. Nr. 5. Mainz: Steiner 1966
10. Gardner, R. J. M.: A new estimate of the achondroplasia mutation rate. Clin. Gent. **11,** 31 1977
11. Herrmann, J., France, T. D., Spranger, J., Opitz, J. M.: The Stickler Syndrome (Hereditary arthroophthalmopathy) Birth Defects. Orig. Art. Series **XI,** No. 2 1975
12. Kopits, S. E.: Orthopedic complications of dwarfism. Clin. Orthop. **114,** 153 1976
13. Kaufmann, E.: Die Chondrodystrophia hyperplastica. Beitr. path. Anat. **13,** 32 1893
14. Ribbing, S.: Studien über hereditäre multiple Epiphysenstörungen. Acta Radiol. Supp. **34,** 1937
15. Müller, W.: Das Bild der multiplen erblichen Störungen der Epiphysenverknöcherung. Z. Orthopäd. **69,** 257 1939
16. Fairbank, K. T.: Dysplasia epiphysialis multiplex. Brit. J. Surg. **34,** 325 1947
17. Meyer, J.: Dysplasia epiphysialis capitis femoris. Acta Orthop. Scand. **34,** 183 1964
18. Thiemann, H.: Juvenile Epiphysenstörungen; idiopathische Erkrankung der Epiphysenknorpel der Fingerphalangen. Fortschr. Röntgen. **14,** 79 1909
19. Bailey, J. A.: Disproportionate Short Stature. Philadelphia: Saunders 1973
20. Larsen, L. J., Schottstaedt, E. R., Bost, F. C.: Multiple congenital dislocations associated with characteristic facial abnormality. J. Pediat. **37,** 574 1950
21. Buxton, S. J. D.: Multiple Deformities in two sisters. Proc. roy. Soc. Med. **32,** 284 1939
22. Rotter, W., Erb, W.: Über eine Systemerkrankung des Mesenchyms mit multiplen Luxationen aus angeborener Gelenkschlaffheit und über Wirbelkörperspalten. Virchows Arch. Path. **316,** 233 1949
23. McKusick, V. A.: Heritable Disorders of Connective Tissue. St. Louis: Mosby 1972
24. Desbuquois, C., Grenier, B., Michel, J., Rossignol, C.: Nanisme chondrodystrophique avec ossification anarchique et polymalformations chez deux soeurs. Arch. Franc. Pédiat. **23,** 573 1966
25. Spranger, J., Langer, L. O.: Spondyloepiphyseal dysplasia congenita. Radiology **94,** 313 1970
26. Pauli, R. M., Madden, J. D., Kranzler, K. J., Culpepper, W., Port, R.: Warfarin therapy initiated during pregnancy and phenotypic chondrodysplasia punctata. J. Pediat. **88,** 506 1976

27. Rimoin, D. L., Silberberg, R., Hollister, D. W.: Chondro-osseous pathology in the chondrodystrophies. Clin. Orthop. **114,** 137 1976

28. Ponseti, I. V.: Skeletal growth in Morquio's disease. In: Zorab, P. A., ed.: Scoliosis and Growth. Edinburgh, London, Churchill Livingstone, 1971

Revised and updated English translation from the German edition *Der Orthopäde,* Vol. 3, pp. 65–71 (1974), Vol. 5, pp. 62–67 (1976), Vol. 5, pp. 75–83 (1976),

Orthopaedic Corrections in Patients with Vitamin D-Resistant Rickets

H. Wagner*

Of the characteristic skeletal deformities caused by vitamin D-resistant rickets in children, the distortions of the long bones of the lower limbs are of major importance from both the functional and the therapeutic points of view.

The following deformities belong to this class (Fig. 1):

Coxa vara
Increased anterior bowing of the femoral shaft
Varus deformity of the femoral shaft
Varus malposition of the femoral condyle
Varus malposition of the proximal tibia
Recurvation of the proximal tibia
Varus deformity of the tibial shaft
Anterior bowing of the tibial shaft

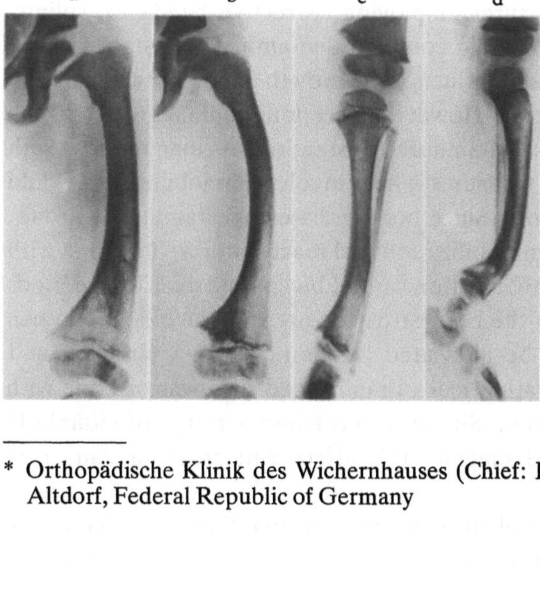

Fig. 1a–d. Typical deformities of vitamin D-resistant rickets. (a) Femur of a 4½-year-old female; varus deformity of the femoral neck; varus deformity with anterior bowing of the shaft at the distal diaphyseal-metaphyseal junction; varus deformity of the femoral condyle. (b) Femur of a 9½-year-old male: a long-arched varus deviation with anterior bowing of the femoral diaphysis; slight varus deformity of the femoral neck; normal femoral condyle. (c) Tibia of a 4½-year-old male: supramalleolar varus deviation with varus deformity of the ankle. (d) Lower leg of a 2½-year-old female: short-arched marked supramalleolar anterior bowing

* Orthopädische Klinik des Wichernhauses (Chief: Prof. Dr. H. Wagner), Nuremberg/Altdorf, Federal Republic of Germany

Supramalleolar varus deformity of the tibia and fibula with or without anterior bowing
Internal rotation deviation of the ankle joint in relation to the axis of the knee joint

In addition, as a result of these malpositions or of disturbed endochondal ossification, one finds shortening of the neck of the femur and dysplasias of the femoral condyle, proximal tibia, patella and ankle mortise.

All these deformities almost always appear symmetrically and may occur individually or in various combinations. Although any metabolic disturbance of the child's skeletal system may cause deformities requiring orthopaedic treatment, vitamin D-resistant rickets represents the most common metabolic disorder necessitating surgery. There are several reasons for this:

Even after very consistent long-term treatment with vitamin D and phosphate, abnormal curvatures of the long bones show only a limited tendency toward spontaneous correction (Branick, Jaffê, Maxwell); there may even be considerable deterioration (Fig. 2). In most patients, pronounced bone deformities are already present when the primary disease is diagnosed. The great extent of the deformity and the markedly asymmetric weight borne by the epiphyseal plates hamper spontaneous straightening. But even if the deformations present at the beginning of treatment are slight, the extent of spontaneous correction is uncertain and must be controlled clinically and roentgenologically.

After instituting treatment there is a distinct improvement of the bone structure in the area of the metaphyses and also in the other bone segments. The considerably widened epiphyseal plate becomes narrower. Increased longitudinal growth of the epiphyses on the concave side of the curvature leads to a diminution of the distortion. However, in contrast to vitamin D-deficiency rickets, a complete normalization cannot be expected.

Conservative orthopaedic measures employing corrective bandages, splints, and other apparatus are of little use in combating vitamin D-resistant rickets. The principle of such treatment is to influence the growth of epiphyseal plates by applying external mechanical forces. However, since longitudinal growth of the epiphyses is slower in patients with vitamin D-resistant rickets than in those with normal metabolisms, corrective measures which involve immobilization would require correspondingly more time. Since bone in cases of vitamin D-resistant rickets is especially sensitive to immobilization and reacts after a short time with severe atrophy of inactivity, immobilization cannot be applied over long periods of time if lasting disturbances to the bone structure are to be avoided. Nor can changes due to immobilization be alleviated by administring vitamin D and mineral supplements. Immobilization leads to enhanced turnover of bone with increased urinary calcium excretion. Simultaneous administration of vitamin D and mineral supplements would magnify this effect and create a danger of nephrocalcinosis.

A still more important problem obstructing conservative therapy is that one is almost always dealing with multiple deformities. The malpositions and distor-

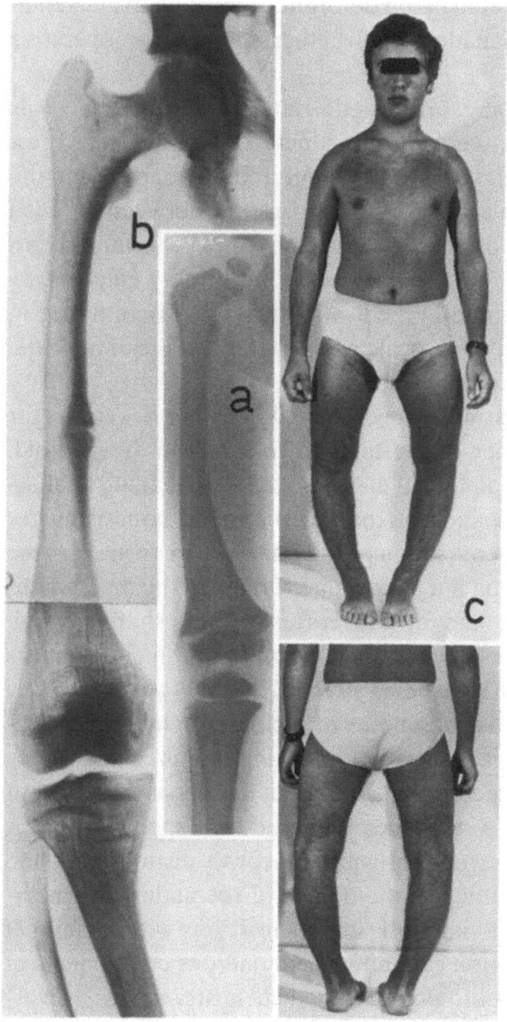

Fig. 2a–c. Increasing deformation of the leg of a now 15-year-old male in spite of continuous vitamin D treatment since age 4 with regular control of serum calcium and phosphate levels and of urinary calcium excretion. (a) Roentgenogram at age 4. (b and c) Status at age 15 (a and b are in scale)

tions previously mentioned are combined in various ways and can, therefore, only appropriately be corrected by operative procedures. Although genu varum may be amenable to conservative treatment, its correction does not take place at the site of the deformity but rather at the site of least resistance or in the area where externally applied forces exert their maximum effect. Thus, for example, it is impossible to correct a varus deformity of the neck of the femur or posterior bowing of the tibia using a plaster cast or other corrective device. The axis of the leg can merely be straightened out in its entirety. In so doing, valgus countercurvatures are created in the distal femoral metaphysis, with persisting, marked varus curvature of the shaft and continuing malposition of the neck of the femur and the proximal tibia.

If no acceptable correction can be expected from the tendency toward spontaneous straightening and the limited possibilities of conservative treatment, then the consequences of the remaining deformities must be evaluated in each individual case and a decision made as to whether an extensive operative correction is justified.

It is self-evident that prior to any orthopaedic intervention, which deals solely with the skeletal deformities, the underlying metabolic disturbance must first be treated by a pediatrician or internist competent in these matters and the patient kept under constant supervision. Close cooperation between surgeon and pediatrician is of decisive importance if surgery is to be considered. An osteotomy will result in an increase in bone turnover and urinary calcium excretion. Therefore, high dosage vitamin D medication must be discontinued in order to prevent hypercalciuria and nephrocalcinosis. After stabilization of the osteotomy, the vitamin D dosage must be recalculated.

The consequences of skeletal deformities in vitamin D-resistant rickets are far reaching. The effects of this disorder of the mineral metabolism are twofold. First, endochondral ossification of epiphyseal plates is inhibited, leading to aberrations in growth; second, mineralization of the newly formed bone is inadequate. This pertains not only to mineralization of the bone matrix formed in the course of physiologic bone remodeling but also to that formed in the metaphyses through endochondral ossification and at the cortex of the shaft through periosteal ossification. This results in weaker bone, a condition which manifests itself primarily in lowered resistance to bending stresses. The metabolic disorder affects the skeleton most severely during phases of increased mineral requirements, that is, during growth and pregnancy and following fractures and osteotomy. The effects are less pronounced during adulthood, but persist throughout life. The bone's mechanical power of resistance is altered correspondingly: It is greatest in adults, but never reaches normal values. Growth disturbances and bone strength vary, of course, according to the degree of the underlying metabolic disorder. Modern treatment of vitamin D-resistant rickets with vitamin D administration and mineral substitution can influence numerous components of the metabolic disorder and even lead to normal blood chemistry values. Nevertheless, clinical experience has shown that it does not guarantee normal mineralization of the skeleton. This is manifested by the inadequate tendency of deformed bones toward spontaneous correction during the growth period and also by the reduced bone strength evident throughout life in patients with vitamin D-resistant rickets.

Orthopaedic Aspects of Vitamin D-Resistant Rickets

Aside from its effects on joint mechanics, the concurrence of distortion and reduced bending strength is an important factor in determining whether surgery is indicated. If the results of clinical and roentgenologic examinations show progressing distortions despite proper treatment of the disorder in the mineral metabolism, it is evident that the bending stresses on the long bones exceed their bending strength and further deformities must be expected (Figs. 2 and 3).

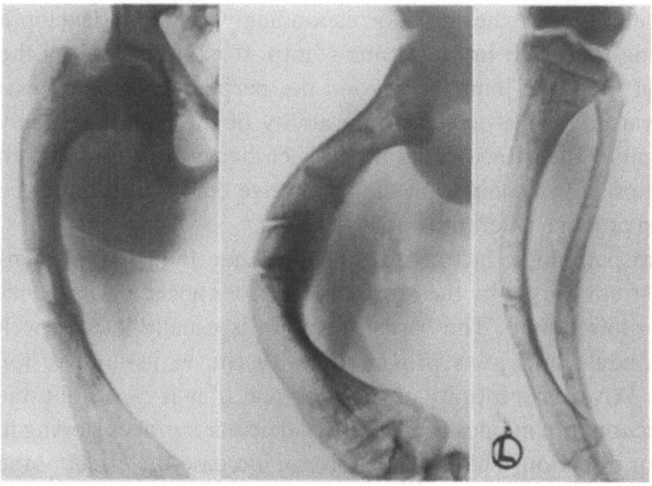

Fig. 3. Excessive bowing of the femur, tibia, and fibula with extreme osteoatrophy and Looser zones in as yet untreated vitamin D-resistant rickets in a 16-year-old male

If Looser zones are ascertainable, it is certain that a marked aggravation of the deformity will occur. In these cases, a corrective osteotomy must be performed without delay. Otherwise the distortions – especially those at the femur – can increase to a point where the patient is no longer able to walk (Fig. 3). It must also be kept in mind that with increasing distortions of the long bones – and this too pertains above all to the thigh – a shortening of the soft tissues on the concave side will occur. Thus, on account of the tension in the soft tissues, a delayed corrective osteotomy can only be carried out by resecting a bone segment. This leads to a shortening of the limb and further reduction of body height. If, on the other hand, the clinical progress examinations show a diminution of the distortion and the mechanical stress factors influencing neighboring joints are favorable, one can await the results of spontaneous correction and, if necessary, carry out the osteotomy at a later date. The results of the correction will be more definitive if it is made near the end of the growth period.

Among the aspects of surgical correction, mechanical stress factors – especially at the hip and knee joints – are of particular importance.

Varus distortion of the neck of the femur is especially common in vitamin D-resistant rickets. In extreme cases, the tip of the greater trochanter lies above the hip joint, and the articular surface of the femoral head is imbedded in the acetabulum in such a manner that the noncartilaginous head-neck transition zone becomes part of the area most under stress. This produces an incongruence of the articular surfaces and thus contributes to the development of osteoarthrosis. Furthermore, the elevated position of the trochanter results in an insufficiency of the pelvitrochanteric musculature. Owing to the internal rotation malposition of the ankle joint, the patient carries his leg in external rotation. This not only intensifies the varus deformity of the knee joint but also turns the usually shortened femoral neck in increased anteversion, further aggravating the musculomechanical conditions at the hip. Correspondingly, patients develop a swaying gait resembling that seen in Duchenne's limp; it is intensified by the lateral displacement of the knee joint far beyond the perpendicular body axis defined by the genu varum. The weight-bearing ability of the limb is severely limited. The interaction of these factors results in such heavy functional strain and such a poor prognosis for the hip joint that operative correction cannot be lightly rejected if it can produce a definite improvement.

The most prominent pathologic factor affecting the knee joint is the asymmetric and abnormal strain caused by the more or less pronounced varus deviation of the axis of the lower limb. The varus deviation is usually located well above the femoral condyle and joins proximally with the varus-anteversion curvature of the shaft. A varus deformity of the proximal tibia is rarer, but one occasionally finds a recurvation malposition with the articular surfaces sloping in an anterior and inferior direction. This recurvation can increase the effect of the genu varum aspect on the weight-bearing limb. In children, the knee joint functions inconspicuously, whereas in juveniles and adults, one can observe a relaxation of the lateral ligamentous apparatus which may well be interpreted as stretch damage. The genu varum is more striking in walking than in standing. This is due partly to the ease with which the lateral interarticular joint spaces open up but is also partly due to the fact that the patient walks with externally rotated legs because of the internal rotation malposition of the ankle joint. Study of the flexed knee joint, in contrast to the clinical appearance in standing, often demonstrates that the lower leg exhibits no varus deformity but rather an internal tibial torsion defect. Nevertheless, defects in vertical alignment may also be observed in the tibial shaft: primarily anterior bowing in the middle third and varus deviations at the transition from the middle to the distal third. The latter add to the more proximally localized deviations and affect the strain on the knee joint. In spite of the various curvatures of the upper and lower legs, the varus stress almost always predominates in the knee joint. This causes no complaints in children but a striking disturbance in gait. On the other hand, in juveniles and adults, it is accompanied by weight-bearing pain. At the medial femoral condyle there occur circumscribed areas of softening which are interpreted biomechanically as fatigue fractures of the subchondral cancellous bone and resemble osteochondrosis dissecans in appearance and significance. Finally, varus gonarthrosis, similar to that seen in malpositions of other origin, arises.

At the distal end of the lower leg, internal rotation malposition of the ankle joint and marked supramalleolar axial angulations are clinically important. The internal tibial torsion of the distal end of the lower leg, not previously described in the literature but present in all of our patients, can vary between 20° and 40°. This deformity is of pathogenetic interest insofar as it is caused by a disorder in the mineral metabolism without a concomitant rotation fault in the growth of an epiphyseal plate. In this connection, it is noteworthy that the normally prismatic profile of the tibia is less clearly defined in vitamin D-resistant rickets; the bone has a rather round cross section. Therefore, one may ask whether these changes are produced by load bearing through forces of torsion acting on weakened bone. But even such a deformation through torsional stress is an unsatisfactory explanation inasmuch as rotation defects are regularly observed in two- to three-year-old children. In any case, it is clinically important to note that rotation defects have a lasting effect on the dynamics of the hip, knee and, ankle joints and almost always develop to a point where correction becomes necessary.

The supramalleolar varus deviation of the leg intensifies the abnormal load on the knee joint but surprisingly causes no complaints in the ankle joint or foot. The varus position of the ankle joint and the compensatory valgus position of the subtalar joint are well tolerated. It is characteristic of most patients with vitamin D-resistant rickets that they have sturdy and meaty feet and rarely complain about them. However, the rare short-arched supramalleolar deviations require correction, as the feet cannot be put down plantigrade and the disturbance in gait is considerable.

Besides the biomechanical and articular dynamics problems, the serious aesthetic disfiguration of patients with vitamin D-resistant rickets should not be ignored. The conspicuous gait and the often grotesque deformities affect the patients' psychologic and social development and impede their vocational advancement. In considering the various methods of therapy, this problem too should be appreciated.

Operative Technique

The goal of operative correction in vitamin D-resistant rickets is to increase the load-bearing capacity of the long bones by correcting the axis and, in so doing, to prevent stress-induced deformities or fatigue fractures. Correction of the joint-forming ends of bones should normalize the requirements of the joints as much as possible and thus check the development of osteoarthrosis. It should also bring about healing of already existing osteochondrotic foci in the knee joint. In improving the load-carrying capacity of the long bones, the load itself is increased, providing an additional mechanical stimulus for bone growth.

As already mentioned, operative treatment should not be undertaken during an active phase of the disease. At least several months of pediatric treatment should precede it, until roentgen examination indicates an improvement of the bone structure, above all of the metaphyses.

Internal fixation is indispensable in correcting vitamin D-resistant rickets. It guarantees accurately defined reconstructions, avoids plaster cast immobilization, and postoperatively enables careful, partial weight-bearing, thereby reducing inactivity atrophy of the bones. Preoperatively, the course and extent of the deformity must be precisely determined. In most cases, standard roentgenograms in two planes do not suffice because the deviations occupy several planes. For example, a standard roentgenogram shows a deformity of the femoral shaft to be less than it actually is because the plane of the deviation is directed anteromedially, i.e., the curvature simultaneously takes a varus and forward direction. Only an oblique view with the ray directed perpendicular to the plane of the curvature will demonstrate the full extent of the deformity. This knowledge is necessary for an accurate correction. Several films may be required for accurate interpretation of the malformation.

Femoral Corrections

Intertrochanteric or Subtrochanteric Valgus Osteotomy

As a separate entity, the varus deformity of the neck of the femur is relatively rare. An intertrochanteric valgus osteotomy with lateral wedge resection is employed for its correction. It can be secured by internal fixation with an angle plate inserted under compression. In inserting the angle plate, utmost care must be taken to preserve the epiphyseal plate of the greater trochanter. Otherwise, there will be growth damage to the proximal end of the femur. Difficulties in internal fixation may occur if for anatomic reasons the length of bone between the trochanteric epiphyseal plate and the osteotomy surface is too short for anchoring the blade of the plate or if the lateral cortex of the proximal fragment is so soft that the blade threatens to tear out under compression. In these cases, the base of the wedge can be placed further distally. This creates a medially upward slanting of the apposed osteotomy surfaces. Fixation with angle plates with a blade-plate angle of 120° permits insertion further distally in the stronger cortical bone. In small children, these stratagems are more difficult. Here the osteotomy can take place just below the lesser trochanter and stabilization can follow comfortably and reliably with a straight plate bent in correspondence to the angle of the osteotomy and fixed to the two fragments with screws (Fig. 4).

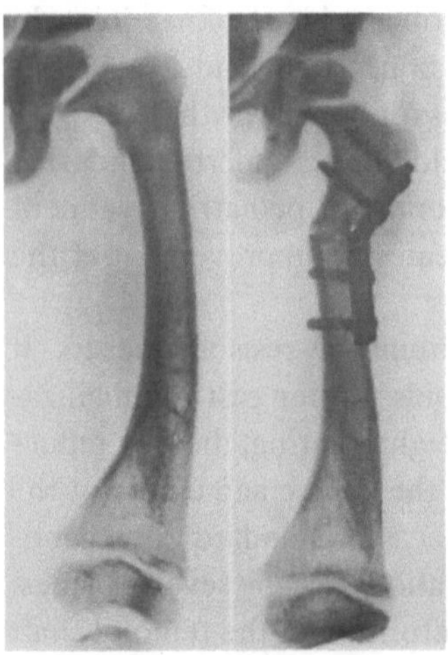

a b

Fig. 4. (a) Coxa vara in a $4^1/_2$-year-old female with vitamin D-resistant rickets. (b) Correction of the femoral neck by subtrochanteric valgus osteotomy and stabilization with a bent, narrow internal fixation plate.

Supracondylar Osteotomy

In the varus deformity of the distal end of the femur, the apex of the curvature is almost always very proximal to the epiphyseal plate. This is a great technical advantage when operating because the osteotomy and internal fixation do not touch the growth zone. In the presence of an open epiphyseal plate, surgery must always be performed in the metaphysis. Stabilizing angle plates can only be used after closure of the epiphyseal plate. In the high supracondylar osteotomy the base of the wedge lies lateral or anterolateral, depending on the course of the curvature. The medial cortex can almost always be left untouched. Owing to the decreased hardness of the bone substance, it remains intact after axial correction. Its tension band effect increases the stability of the site of internal fixation. For stabilization of the osteotomy, application of a T-plate or hook plate suffices. However, should the medial cortex have to be transected, e.g., should it be necessary to displace the proximal fragments medially, one can secure the medial osteotomy cleft by a lag screw inserted diagonally.

Diaphyseal Femoral Osteotomy

In the majority of cases involving the femur, a combination of deformities is present. Malpositions of the femoral neck and femoral condyle are found together with deviations of the femoral shaft. This poses special technical problems for operative correction. Theoretically, an ideal correction of a combination deformity would call for several osteotomies carried out at various levels. Out of practical, clinical considerations, however, such a serial segmental resection of the femur is generally not feasible. Preferably, the operation should be carried out at the apex of the deformities and all malpositions be corrected at the same time at one point. Following exact roentgen localization of the course of the deviation, the optimal level for osteotomy is ascertained by preoperative construction tracings. This problem can be solved satisfactorily in most cases by a diaphyseal wedge osteotomy. For stabilization, a straight osteosynthesis plate is inserted under pressure and bent to the desired angle of correction. Following wedge osteotomy, the diaphyseal fragments are brought into apposition with slight overcorrection and the metal plate is applied to the osteotomy site. Owing to the overcorrection of the fragments, the ends of the plate rest on the bone. Its midportion does not touch the bone at the height of the osteotomy. The ends of the plate are screwed onto the bone and then, working toward the middle, the remaining screws are inserted. When the screws are tightened, the diaphyseal fragments are drawn closer to the plate whereby they become relatively longer and put tension on the plate (Fig. 5). The stability of the fixation is thus substantially increased. If the diaphyseal osteotomy lies exactly in the middle of the femur, the effect of the correction is divided equally between the upper and lower ends of the femur. If the osteotomy is performed at a more cranial or caudal site, the correction of either the femoral neck or femoral condyle, respectively, is more pronounced (Fig. 6). The original postoperative angulation of the femoral shaft straightens itself in the course of time through bone accumulation on the concave side and bone removal on the convex side.

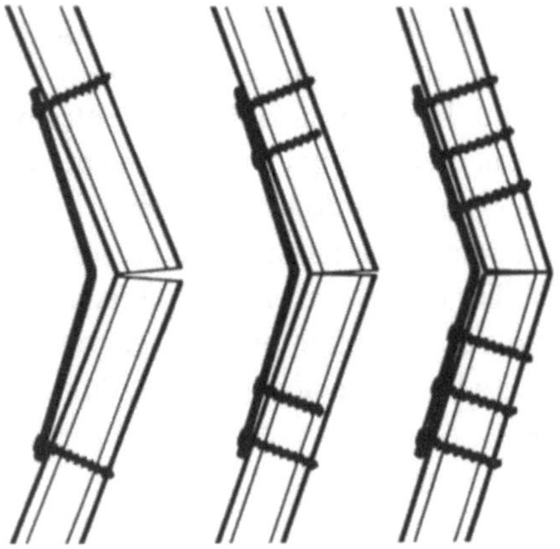

Fig. 5. Diaphyseal femoral osteotomy. Stabilization with bent internal fixation plate. The fragments are apposed with slight overcorrection and the plate placed over the osteotomy site. Due to overcorrection of the fragments, the ends of the plate are in contact with the bone while the middle portion is raised from it at the level of the osteotomy. The plate is secured to the bone with screws, working from its ends to the middle. When the screws are tightened, the fragments are drawn to the plate whereby they become relatively longer and place the plate under tension

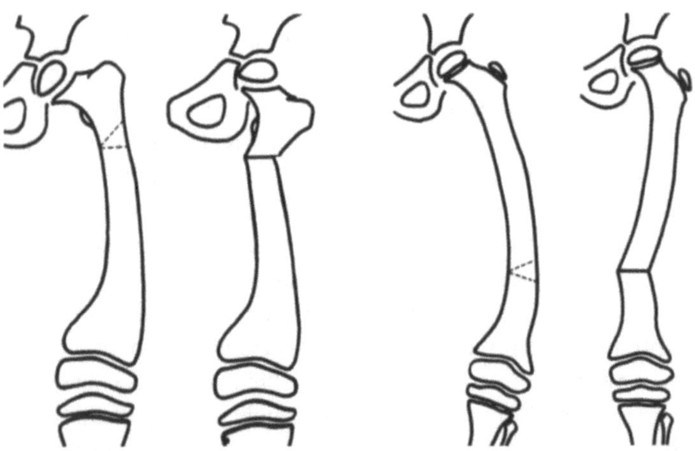

Fig. 6. Diaphyseal femoral osteotomy for correction of a varus deformity of the femoral neck and condyle and varus deviation of the shaft. If the osteotomy site lies at the middle of the femur, the correction is equally effective at both ends. If it is more cranial, correction is more pronounced at the femoral neck and vice versa

Proximal Tibial Osteotomy

To protect the apophyseal growth plate and to ensure reliable internal fixation, the proximal tibial osteotomy should be done distal to the tuberosity of the tibia. The operation should be preceded by an osteotomy of the fibula to avoid obstruction. The oblique osteotomy of the fibula at the transition from the pro-

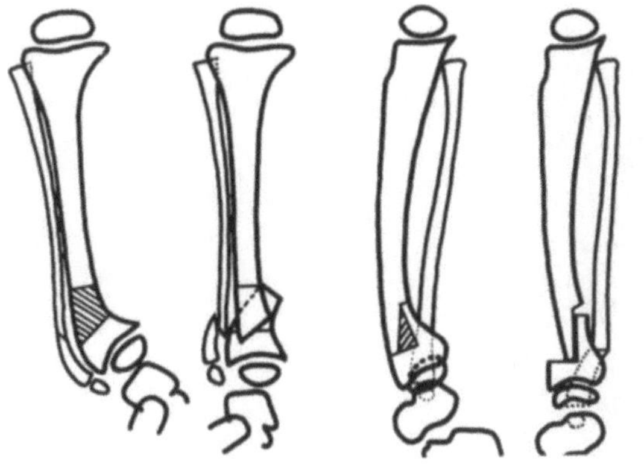

Fig. 7. Supramalleolar osteotomy. The stepcut osteotomy is carried out in the frontal plane. By turning the distal fragments in the osteotomy surface, the varus curvature is corrected. Removal of a bone wedge in the frontal plane with a distal base at the same time permits correction of a supramalleolar anterior bowing

ximal to the middle third is simple and well-established; bone consolidation takes place quickly because the fragments remain in contact.

For correction of a varus deformity of the proximal tibia, a lateral wedge osteotomy is carried out. A base of 3–5 mm is adequate in most cases. The medial cortex does not have to be osteomized and a T-plate applied laterally under tension provides sufficient stabilization. It is easier to employ a narrow hook plate if the cross section of the bone is small. If, in addition to the osteotomy of the proximal tibia, a recurvation or rotation defect must be corrected or if a displacement of the fragments in the lateral plane is necessary, osteotomy of the medial cortex must also be carried out. For stabilization, a diagonally applied lag screw or a medially applied small compression plate is then required.

a b

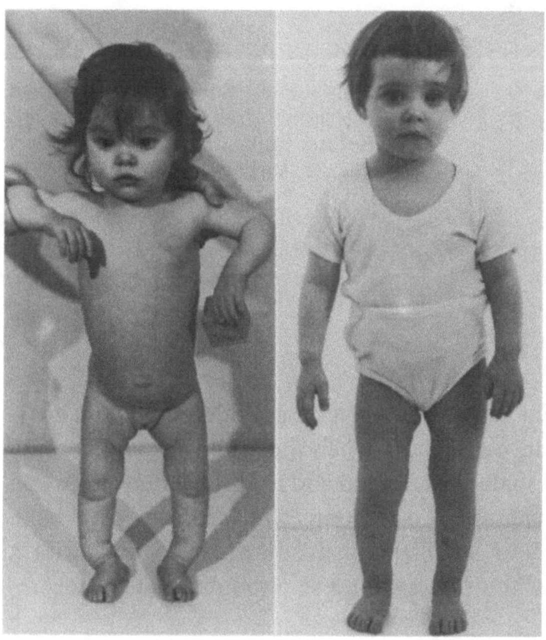

Fig. 8 a and b. Bilateral supramalleolar tibial osteotomy in a $2^1/_2$-year-old female with vitamin D-resistant rickets. Before (a) and $1^1/_2$ years after (b) surgery

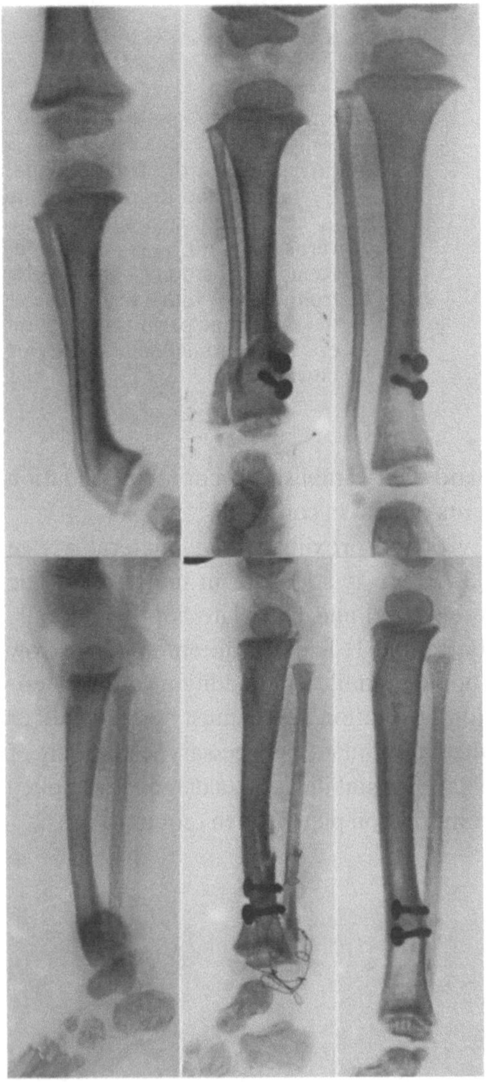

a b c

Fig. 9a–c. Supramalleolar tibial osteotomy (same case as Fig. 8). Before (a), at (b), and $1^1/_2$ years after (c) surgery

Diaphyseal Tibial Osteotomy

As in the femur, diaphyseal tibial osteotomy must be considered when a combination of deformities is present, particularly when a marked varus deformity and anterior bowing of the tibial shaft exists. Axial and rotational deviations can be corrected by a transverse diaphyseal osteotomy with removal of a bone wedge of the appropriate size. For stabilization, fixation of the tibia with a narrow compression plate and of the fibula with a semitubular plate is recommended.

Supramalleolar Osteotomy

The supramalleolar osteotomy is indicated in the rare, short-arched, supramalleolar angulations of the leg. Because of the special anatomic circumstances

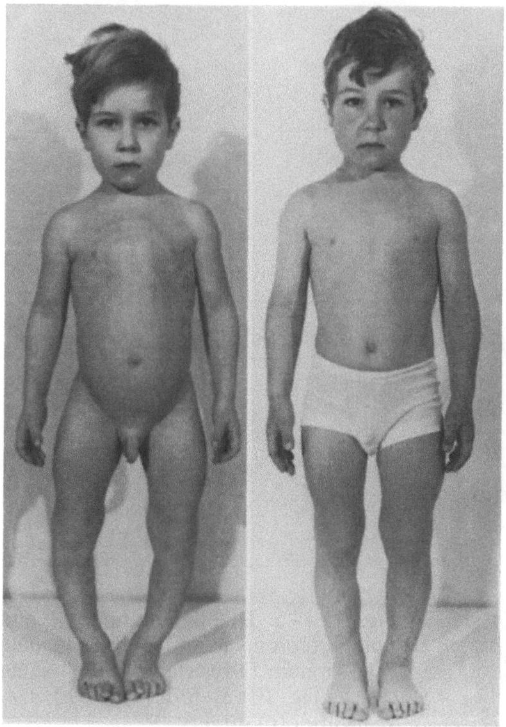

a b

Fig. 10a and b. Bilateral diaphyseal femoral and tibial osteotomy in a $5^1/_2$-year-old male with vitamin D-resistant rickets. Before (a) and $1^1/_2$ years after (b) surgery

which make osteotomy – especially internal fixation – difficult, we have found the stepcut frontal osteotomy to be useful. It allows for corrections of sufficient magnitude and yet retains extensive contact between the surfaces of the fragments. This is beneficial for the fixation and bone consolidation. The fragments of the supramalleolar osteotomy are stabilized with small lag screws, either singly or in combination with a semitubular plate. If necessary, a plaster walking cast may be applied to the lower leg (Figs. 7–9).

Summary

The characteristic and often very serious deformities of the long bones in vitamin D-resistant rickets, especially those involving the lower extremity, require operative treatment. Chemotherapy of the underlying disorder of mineral

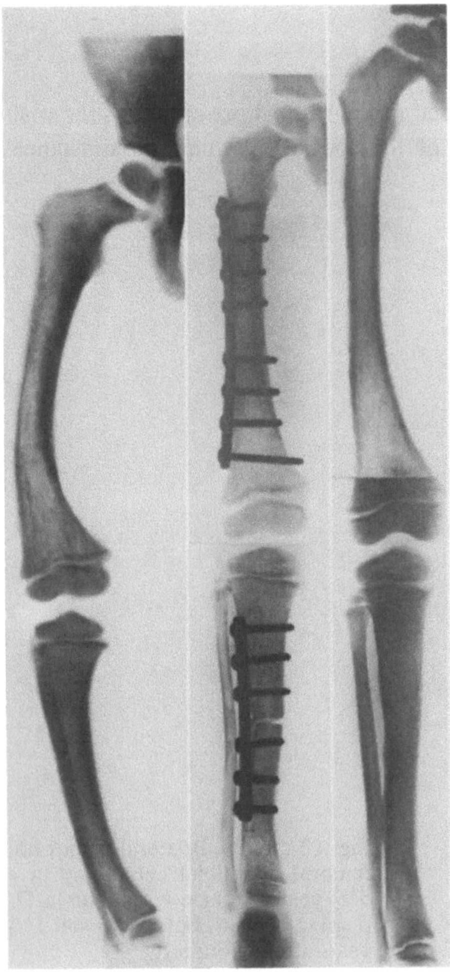

a b c

Fig. 11 a–c. Diaphyseal femoral and tibial osteotomy in a $5^1/_2$-year-old male with vitamin D-resistant rickets (same case as Fig. 10). Before (a), at (b), $1^1/_2$ years after (c) surgery

metabolism alone does not foster an adequate spontaneous correction. The most extensive correction possible is necessary. Otherwise, as a result of reduced bone strength, stress deformities will occur which are not amenable even to vigorous chemotherapy and which can lead to considerable disfigurement and disorders in gait. Today, stable internal fixation enables extensive reconstruction and lessens inactivity atrophy of the bone to a tolerable extent.

In general, experience with corrective surgery in vitamin D-resistant rickets is still very limited. In our clinic, 36 such operative corrections have been carried out in the past 7 years. Observation to date show that accurate surgical correct-

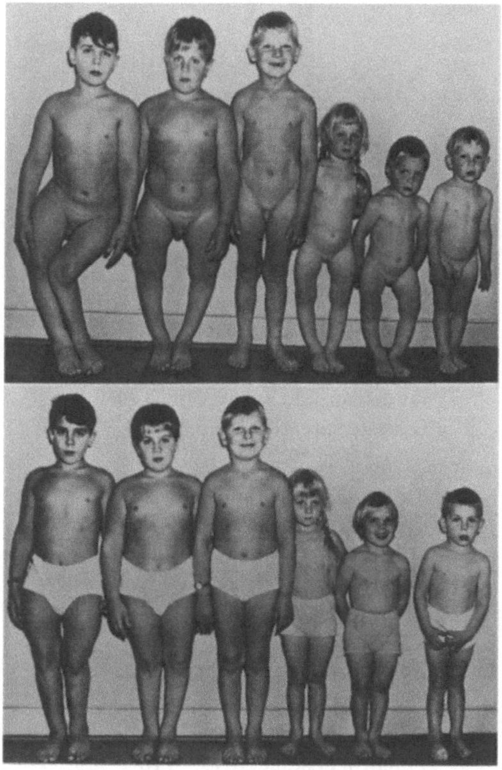

Fig. 12. Six siblings, four of them affected by vitamin D-resistant rickets. Before (a) and 2 years after (b) surgery

ion together with chemotherapy can prevent recurring deformities. Thus far, we have not had to reoperate on any patients. An absolute prerequisite for successful treatment is careful supervision and medical management of the underlying metabolic disorder by the pediatrician before and after operation.

References

Branick, R. L.: J. Bone Jt Surg. **50-A,** 1062 (1968)
Jaffê, H. L.: Metabolic, Degenerative and Inflammatory Diseases of Bones and Joints. Philadelphia: Lea & Febiger 1972
Maxwell, C. M.: J. Bone Jt Surg. **54-B,** 202 (1972)

English translation from the German edition *Der Orthopäde,* Vol. 3, pp. 91–99 (1974),

Subject Index

List of Contributors

Dega, Prof. Dr. W.
Dzierzyńskiego 135, 61–545 Poznań, Poland

G. D. MacEwen, M. D.
Alfred I. DuPont Institute, P. O. Box 269, Wilmington, Delaware 19899, USA

Morscher, Prof. Dr. E.
Orthopädische Universitäts-Klinik, Felix-Platter-Spital, Burgfelderstraße 101, CH-4005 Basel, Switzerland

H. L. Moss, M. D.
Departments of Surgery (Orthopaedics) and Pediatrics, and Human Growth and Development Study Unit, Yale University School of Medicine, New Haven, Connecticut 06510, USA

J. A. Ogden, M. D.
Departments of Surgery (Orthopaedics) and Pediatrics, and Human Growth and Development Study Unit, Yale University School of Medicine, New Haven, Connecticut 06510, USA

Schuster, Prof. Dr. W.
Röntgenabteilung Pädiatrie, Klinikum der Justus-Liebig-Universität, Feulgenstraße 12, D-6300 Gießen, Federal Republic of Germany

Spranger, Prof. Dr. J.
Klinikum der Johannes-Gutenberg-Universität, Kinderklinik, Langenbeckstraße 1, D-6500 Mainz, Federal Republic of Germany

D. C. Stephens, M. D.
Alfred I. DuPont Institute, P. O. Box 269, Wilmington, Delaware 19899, USA

Strauß, Dr. J.
Orthopädische Klinik des Wichernhauses, Postfach 22, D-8503 Altdorf, Federal Republic of Germany

Wagner, Prof. Dr. H.
Orthopädische Klinik des Wichernhauses, Postfach 22, D-8503 Altdorf, Federal Republic of Germany

Progress in Orthopaedic Surgery

Volume 1

Leg Length Discrepancy The Injured Knee

Editor: D. S. Hungerford

With contributions by W. Bandi, J. Eichler, G. Figner, P. Heidensohn, E. Hogue, D. Hohmann, J. L. Hughes, C. Kieser, E. Meyer, E. Morscher, W. Müller, D. Petersen, A. Rüttimann, H. Wagner, M. Weigert

100 figures. X, 160 pages. 1977
ISBN 3-540-08037-6

Contents:

Leg Length Discrepancy:
Baisc Rehabilitation Principles of Persons with Leg Length Discrepancy: An Overview. – Etiology and Pathopyhsiology of Leg Length Discrepancies. – Measurement of Leg Length. – Methodological Errors in Documenting Leg Length and Leg Length Discrepancies. – Equalization of Leg Length with Orthopaedic Shoe Measures. – Subtrochanteric Shortening and Lengthening Osteotomy. – Surgical Lengthening or Shortening of Femur and Tibia. Technique and Indications.
The Injured Knee:
The Importance of Arthography Following Trauma to the Knee Joint. – The Knee Joint of the Soccer Player (Its Stresses and Damages). – Trauma-Induced Chondromalacia Patellae. – Traumatic Injuries to the Articular Cartilage of the Knee. – Subject Index. – List of Contributors.

Foreword

Two timely topics have been selected by the editors for the initial volume of the new series *Progress in Orthopaedic Surgery*.
The series begins with primarily European contributions on a subject which is more prevalent in Europe than in many of the English speaking countries. It is therefore not surprising that significant advances have been achieved in the evaluation and treatment of significant leg length discrepancy based on the need to solve the associated complex technical problems. This section on leg length discrepancy comprehensively covers the problem from diagnosis, methods of quantifying discrepancy, and pathomechanics to non-surgical and surgical treatment of the discrepancy. Recognized experts in the field have concisely presented their experience. Together these articles comprise a section which represents the "state of the art" for evaluation and treatment of leg length discrepancy. The second topic deals with the injured knee. Dr. Müller presents comprehensive overview of the soccer player's knee. With the growing interest and involvement of this sport in the United States involving all age groups, this article will be particularly appreciated.
Professors Bandi and Wagner deal with the question of cartilage injury in the knee. Certainly such lesions occur more frequently than they are diagnosed. Professor Bandi brings his longstanding interest and experience in patella pathology to bear on the question of a traumatic etiology of chondromalacia patellae. Professor Wagner elucidates a variety of kinds of cartilage injury, both direct and indirect, with practical suggestions for diagnosis and treatment.
This first issue of *Progress in Orthopaedic Surgery* has been edited to introduce English-speaking orthopaedists to the works and thinking of their German-speaking colleagues. Outstanding work on timely topics has been selected with the hope that this series will provide a common ground for communication between these two important language groups.

David S. Hungerford, M. D.

MIX
Papier aus verantwortungsvollen Quellen
Paper from responsible sources
FSC® C105338

If you have any concerns about our products,
you can contact us on
ProductSafety@springernature.com

In case Publisher is established outside the EU,
the EU authorized representative is:
Springer Nature Customer Service Center GmbH
Europaplatz 3, 69115 Heidelberg, Germany

Printed by Libri Plureos GmbH
in Hamburg, Germany